Treatment Planning for Rehabilitation:
A Patient-Centered Approach

Treatment Planning for Rehabilitation: A Patient-Centered Approach

Mark N. Ozer, M.D.
Professor, Department of Neurology
Georgetown University Medical School
Director, Program for Clinical Excellence
National Rehabilitation Hospital
Washington, D.C.

Otto D. Payton, Ph.D., PT, FAPTA
Professor of Physical Therapy
School of Allied Health Professions
Medical College of Virginia
Virginia Commonwealth University
Richmond, Virginia

Craig E. Nelson, M.S., OTR
Occupational Therapy and Rehabilitative Services Director
Hiram W. Davis Medical Center
Petersburg, Virginia

McGraw-Hill
Health Professions Division
New York • St. Louis • San Francisco • Auckland • Bogotá • Caracas • Lisbon • London
Madrid • Mexico City • Milan • Montreal • New Delhi • San Juan
Singapore • Sydney • Tokyo • Toronto

McGraw-Hill

A Division of The **McGraw-Hill** Companies

Treatment Planning for Rehabilitation:
A Patient-Centered Approach

First edition published as *Patient Participation in Program Planning* by
F. A. Davis, © 1990.

1234567890 DOCDOC 99

ISBN 0-07-077882-5

This book was set in Garamond by Better Graphics, Inc.
The editors were Stephen Zollo and Peter McCurdy;
the production supervisor was Catherine Saggese;
The cover was designed by Mary McDonnell.
The index was prepared by Jerry Ralya.
R. R. Donnelley and Sons was printer and binder.

This book is printed on acid-free paper.

Cataloging-in-Publication Data is on file for this title at the Library of Congress.

To Mallory
C.N.

and

To Sam and Max
M.N.O.

Contents

PREFACE

This book is designed for use by students in physical and occupational therapy and by therapists in the course of in-service training. It is designed so that the reader can continue training by self-study. The final goal of this educational program is to be able to demonstrate the knowledge and skills needed to involve patients and clients in a fruitful and productive way in the management of their own therapeutic program.

The method for involving patients in planning arose from my experience with a large variety of persons with disabilities. The adaptation of these methods to physical and occupational therapy and the development of methods for educating professionals in those fields came about in conjunction with my colleagues in writing this book as we worked with students over many years.

The earlier version of this book reflected work with a series of courses for students in physical and occupational therapy at undergraduate, graduate, and in-service levels of training. As the courses developed, they involved many students over the years. Each group of students provided insights and made contributions to the focus of our work. One instance of such contribution is that all the examples used in this book are real-life situations experienced by the students or clinicians in the use of the methods described.

It has been gratifying that the first edition of this book met with considerable praise and was used in a variety of settings. Research traditions were begun in several university-level therapy programs leading to numerous publications in referred journals with students participating as co-authors. Training institutes were presented at state and national professional meetings with positive responses. Most particularly, the process has been used at the National Rehabilitation Hospital in Washington, D.C. and the Medical College of Virginia, Virginia Commonwealth University, and other settings where there has been the opportunity to develop a wider range of examples of clinical application and therefore expand the scope of this second edition. We recognize the contributions of many therapists as well as nurses, psychologists, and other professional staff over the years who have brought the methods to new levels of implementation. Particularly note-worthy have been the contributions of Fatemah Milani, M.D., and Bren-dan Conroy, M.D., physicians on the Stroke Recovery Program at the National Rehabilitation Hospital, and the work of Paul Rao, Ph.D., who was the co-director of that program. We dedicate this book to the numerous students and clinicians who have worked with the principles to bring them to life. The hope is that these individuals will continue to use the ideas exemplified in this book to grow in their professional lives by helping their clients perfect their own skills.

Mark N. Ozer, M.D.

Treatment Planning for Rehabilitation:
A Patient-Centered Approach

Part 1

The Planning Process

Within this first section of principles, the format of the book replicates the planning process it illustrates. The planning process starts with the identification of a problem, then the description of methods for solution followed by the setting of goals. Using this same order, the first chapter (The Overall Plan) deals with issues or problems in the field of rehabilitation that the book is designed to alleviate, with general methodologic principles and the goals of the book. By the end of this chapter, the reader can use the exercise, Planning for Oneself I, to put into practice the planning process by addressing the problems suggested in the chapter. The problems can be those arising in one's own educational activity in performing the procedures described in this book. They can also be those

1

developing at the administrative level in eventually creating a plan for implementation of the procedures to be described.

The remainder of this first section deals with the procedures by which the problems identified in the field of rehabilitation can be alleviated by use of this book. The second chapter (The Planning Process) describes the planning questions one asks and the steps used to answer them. By the end of this chapter, the reader can use the exercise, Planning for Oneself II, to complete the initial planning process for one's own educational plan by addressing the question as to goals in relation to the concerns defined in the earlier exercise at the end of Chapter 1. The third chapter (The Patient as Participant) completes the description of the planning process. It focuses on the degree to which the primary participant (patient or family) is able to participate in answering the planning questions. Increasing the degree of participation can enhance the appropriateness of the answers. Concomitantly, such participation can increase the commitment of energy to the implementation of the plans so generated.

By initiating the planning process in the earlier exercises, there is now an opportunity in the exercise entitled Planning for Oneself III to review and evaluate the outcome of one's own education plan and the means by which goals were accomplished. Figure I-1 illustrates this process by which you (reader/student) in interaction with the instructor can begin to perform your own planning process.

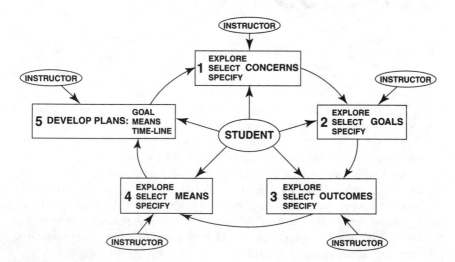

Figure I-1. Student participation in educational planning.

2

By the end of these chapters describing the procedures in their entirety, the reader can put them into practice and devise an initial planning activity with a patient. The exercise entitled Application to Patient Care I reflects this activity. One should be aware of the use of the planning questions and the degree to which the patient is able to participate. Readers can also evaluate their own abilities in performing the procedures for the first time with patients in actual application and recycle the planning process initiated at the start of this section. Figure I-2 illustrates the cycle you are now entering in relation to your patients, analogous to that you have just undergone in relation to your instructor and the material provided in Part One.

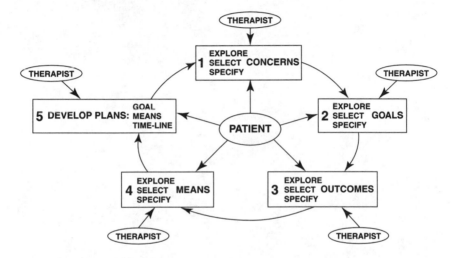

Figure I-2.   Patient participation in program planning.

Chapter 1
The Overall Plan

WHAT IS THE PROBLEM?

WHAT WOULD WORK?
Standards
Models
Evidence

WHAT IS THE GOAL?

APPLICATION TO ONESELF I
What Are My Concerns?

WHAT IS THE PROBLEM?

The issue of patient "adherence" to instructions given by health professionals is a serious problem. The usual terms used, "compliance" or "noncompliance," betray an approach to patient care that is perhaps a major part of the problem. These terms infer a relationship in which the patient is under orders to perform. This book suggests that the character of the interaction between the patient as a client and the professional be reconsidered to reflect a sharing of information and responsibility. The problem in failing to carry out regimens will be seen as one that is shared by both parties in the interaction and not the responsibility of the patient alone.

DiMatteo and DiNicola (1) have provided a detailed summary and discussion of the literature on patient compliance with prescribed treatment regimens. Subsequent literature has only confirmed their conclusions. The news is not good. Patients follow a physician's instructions less than 50% of the time if treatment is aimed at long-term prevention. The percentage following instructions is considerably higher (about 75%) if treatment is directed to relieve signs and symptoms of concern to the patient. Although most studies have dealt with the use of medication, some investigations have examined patient follow-through with exercise programs and other behavior recommendations of health practitioners other than physicians. Dishman and colleagues (2) have estimated that 50% of those who start general exercise programs discontinue them within 6 months. On the other hand, knowing that there would be a re-evaluation increased long-term follow-through (12 weeks) to an exercise program (3).

Similar studies have dealt with the usage of equipment prescribed by occupational therapists. In a follow-up study, Allen found that only 43% of persons with quadriplegia continued to use their wrist-driven flexor hinge splint (4). Others have found that 60% of persons with rheumatoid arthritis carried out a prescribed splint program (5). Considerably more successful was the use of adaptive equipment by persons who had undergone hip arthroplasty. The largest percentage of persons used their equipment "always." This success was attributed to the use of a thorough assessment procedure, but it may be noted that the therapist and the patient jointly set postdischarge goals (6).

Noncompliance often leads to less than optimum therapeutic outcomes to the detriment of both the patient and health care professional. The problems leading to noncompliance are multiple (7), not the least of which is miscommunication. Noncompliance also carries ethical implications (8). Some of these problems may diminish with greater patient participation and investment in program planning and outcomes assessment. The importance of confronting this problem is its effect on the outcomes, including costs, of health care. Failure to follow through with plans may jeopardize the person's health as well as the effectiveness of treatment. Lack of adherence to recommendations also interferes with research intended to determine the efficacy of treatments.

Part of the problem may be attributed to the incongruity between the goals stated by patients and those of their therapists (9). In a rehabilitation unit of a general hospital, the patients tended to have such functional goals as "walking," whereas the therapist's goals were often stated in physiologic terms such as "increased strength in the quadriceps muscle." When one compared treatment goals set by occupational therapists with those indicated by patients, there was frequent lack of agreement as to treatment goals of persons with quadriplegia (10).

> The foundation of care given by practitioners is the relationship between the practitioner and the patient, a relationship vitally important to both. This relationship is a medium for the exchange of all forms of information, feelings, and concerns, a factor in the success of therapeutic regimens, and an essential ingredient in the satisfaction of both patient and practitioner. For patients, the relationship with their provider frequently is the most therapeutic aspect of the health care encounter (11).

It therefore becomes critical for both educators and practitioners to focus on the quality of these relationships (12).

The current focus of third-party payers and governmental agencies is on the need to make health care, including rehabilitation, more cost effective. As various techniques for accomplishing cost reduction are tried, the need remains to maintain the quality of outcomes achieved as much as possible. Given the evidence cited earlier in this chapter, one reasonable approach is to enlist the ideas and perceptions of the persons most intimately involved—the person with the injury or illness and the personal caregiver. Ways need to be found to make the client and family or significant caregivers contributing members of the treatment team. By enlisting their ideas, one can also increase their commitment of time and energy—adherence—thus enhancing the effectiveness of the professional staff, making treatment more cost effective. Patient adherence to treatment recommendations is one of the critical components of optimal outcomes. The objective must be to work smarter rather than harder.

The philosophical goal of any rehabilitation program must be to increase the ability of individuals to manage their own lives in the context of ongoing disability to the greatest extent possible. This same principle motivates the movement toward independent living. It is often the responsibility of health care personnel to teach the techniques of self-management during the rehabilitation training process. Such training should ideally begin by empowering the individual to take a meaningful role in planning the rehabilitation program itself (13). A functional outcome or goal can be defined as something that someone else will have to do to or for clients if the clients cannot do it for themselves (14). If clients cannot feed or dress themselves or earn a living, someone will have to do it for them; this is not true if they cannot do full range of motion or lift 10 pounds with their right quadriceps.

The making of the rehabilitation plan and its ongoing review and revision is a basic process in the treatment of any problem. The planning process can be the place where the person with disabilities can learn the skills that will frequently be necessary for the rest of one's life. By involving the client in the rehabilitation process, both the initial active stage of rehabilitation and the rest of the person's life may be optimized. The client can be led to see the rehabilitation process as an opportunity to regain control of one's body and life after injury. Experiencing such control over one's treatment is the site for learning important new skills necessary for the future (15). In subsequent chapters a method will be presented for training health care professionals to make patients their partners in the rehabilitative endeavor.

Patients develop a rich language for describing the sensation, awareness, and meanings of pain, which is often at odds with the mind set of the health care system (16). Incongruity often results when the therapist concentrates on the anatomic/physiologic/kinesiologic level of **impairment** while the patient focuses on the **disability** resulting from such an impairment (17–19). For example, the same objective impairment resulting from an injury to the hand produces far different disabilities in a radio announcer than in a pianist. One should consider not only the degree of objective impairment but the interaction of that impairment with the person, his or her history and goals, and the environment in which that person seeks to function (20).

Given this lack of congruity, many patients may not see the relevance of the therapeutic program to their goals, and so participation is compromised. The understanding of communications by many patients is very concrete, to the extent that they see no connection between their felt needs and the statements of therapists (21). Measurement of the degree of accomplishment of the goals by patients is also more likely if the goals are stated in terms within the patient's experience. Such participation by patients in the process of assessment of the accomplishment of goals helps them expend the effort necessary for continued success; it helps them cope (22).

Conversely, the patient's contribution to goal setting may lack the precision or specificity necessary for adequate delineation of either the problem or the goal. Rogers and Figone studied the life goals of persons with quadriplegia who were at least 1 year postdischarge. They found that most of their subjects were not following established goals and that they lacked the ability to develop goals for themselves (23). One interpretation is that these patients were not taught how to take care of themselves during their initial rehabilitation (24).

Clearly, for various reasons, some patients are not capable of taking an active role in their planning, even when essential facts have been clearly explained to them. In such cases, the health professional does what is legally and ethically best for the patients. In taking such a role, the health professional must understand the limited commitment thus made by these patients to their own care. The problem is how to enable these patients to participate to the greatest degree possible in planning and evaluating their treatment plan and, thus, take an equivalent active role in the ongoing implementation of the plan—to commit the energy to make success more likely. The therapist must do everything possible to help the clients assume responsibility, that is, to speak for themselves as a prerequisite to acting for themselves. One may optimize treatment outcomes and demonstrate the efficacy of treatment.

Issues of compliance, patient participation, and assumption of responsibility are not merely theoretical ones. Therapists in practice were asked about the relevance of these issues to their daily work with clients. These therapists emphasized that they perceived patient participation to be at the core of the way health professionals seek to function. Additionally, the need for patient participation could be a means of dealing with the important issue of staff "burnout."

The problem, then, that this book addresses is how to create more effective collaboration in planning between the patient and the therapist. The goals must arise from the patient to the maximal extent possible, consistent with making those goals clear, specific, and operational. Only the patient can ultimately determine whether a goal is worth the effort. It is the patient who must expend the energy if the goal is to be accomplished. Therefore, the core content of the goal must come from the patient and must be stated in terms the patient can understand. If this is accomplished during the planning process, then the term "compliance" ceases to be appropriate. Compliance infers obedience to rules and regulations, to instructions given. It would be more useful to invite the person to become a collaborative partner to the extent possible. The therapist is thus operating at the level of making recommendations or offering suggestions rather than giving orders. Working with a therapeutic plan made with the patient's participation then becomes an act

of freedom and responsibility for the patient rather than one of obedience, compliance, or even adherence.

WHAT WOULD WORK?

Standards

The *Evaluative Criteria for Accreditation of Education Programs for the
Preparation of Physical Therapists* (25) requires that graduates involve
patients in goal setting, promote interpersonal relationships, demonstrate effective oral communication, and provide psychosocial support
to their patients. These skills are prerequisite to obtaining informed consent (26), and the American Physical Therapy Association standards (27)
require that therapists obtain informed consent for treatment from their
patients. The patient's informed consent requires the patient's rational
participation in decision-making about his or her own care (28).

A comparable sequence of standards is in place for the development of knowledge and skills that will lead to informed consent as an
integral part of patient care (29–31). Similar support can be found in the
accreditation standards for hospitals and rehabilitation facilities and in
the medical literature (32,33). In recognition of these issues, the Code
of Ethics for Occupational Therapy emphasizes a concern for the welfare and dignity of the recipient of services. Among the criteria are that
the persons served be included in the treatment planning process and
that goal-directed services be provided. Patient participation is thus now
recognized as essential to the delivery of high-quality care and is incorporated as a factor in the evaluation of various rehabilitation facilities
and services (34,35).

Models

Do we have a theoretical foundation for attempting to implement these
standards? Perhaps theory is too precise a word for the current level of
development of the research in the literature, but at least we have a
couple of workable conceptual models.

The term **conceptual model** is used to represent a paradigm that
is based on theory or is a precursor to theory. Whereas a theory typi-
cally consists of a statement or a series of statements concerning the
complex interrelationships among concepts (36,37), a conceptual model
offers a contextual framework within which one may organize specific
observations of phenomena. This guides one's thinking and may lead

to further observations or investigations that might not otherwise occur. Second, a conceptual model helps to generate hypotheses that may be tested empirically. By testing hypotheses, researchers can test the extent to which theoretical or conceptual propositions hold true under the specific circumstances of the study. Finally, conceptual models can create within people a way of seeing and understanding the world around them. They can help people to recognize and interpret significant interactions among people and phenomena; they can help to identify causality. Having the ability to shape the world-view of individuals, conceptual models can also, unfortunately, bias observations, by leading one toward conclusions that fit the model, when in fact, the observations may be interpreted by another more accurate model.

Both Engels and Dean have provided conceptual models for organizing observations about patient behavior and a way of seeing and understanding significant interactions between therapists and patients. Engel has written that physicians are greatly influenced by the conceptual model they use to organize their knowledge about patients and their problems; he compares the results of using a biopsychosocial model with using the traditional biomedical model (38,39).

The biomedical model is based on the biologic sciences with diagnosis as its capstone. The newer biopsychosocial model attempts to account for the human experience of the diagnosis as perceived by the client or patient. In the earlier paper, Engel stated, "Establishing a relationship between particular biochemical processes and the clinical data of illness requires a scientifically rational approach to behavioral and psychosocial data, for these are the terms in which most clinical phenomena are reported by patients" (38). He noted that treating the biochemical problem often does not restore "health." The biopsychosocial model attempts to explain the experience of illness, not just the diagnosis of disease.

As Tresolini (11) has pointed out, the relationship between the health care provider and the patient must be based on a shared understanding of the meaning of the patient's illness or impairment if their relationship is to be therapeutic. The biopsychosocial matrix does not refer to three separate entities but to the experiences of one integrated person. Sadler and Hulgus have noted that problems of knowledge, ethics, and pragmatics must all be addressed to apply the biopsychosocial model successfully (40).

In the second paper, Engel (39) gives an example of the application of the biopsychosocial model to a patient with an acute myocardial infarction. Other examples of the application of this model may be found in the literature. Waddell has applied the model to the treatment of low-back pain from a physician's perspective (41) and Dworkin and

Massoth have applied it to the dentist's treatment of temporomandibu-lar disorders (42).

Elizabeth Dean proposed a model for physical therapy practice that postulated optimal treatment outcomes as resulting from an interaction between psychobiologic factors associated with the patient and profes-sional factors associated with the therapist (43). Her model provides constructs for a comprehensive model of practice that includes four primary psychobiologic factors (anatomy, physiology, pathology, psy-chology) with four secondary psychosocial factors (occupation/envi-ronment, life-style, stress management, sociology) in the patient's profile. In the therapist's profile she discussed four primary clinical fac-tors (therapeutic techniques, modalities, patient education, prevention) with four secondary professional factors (two levels in both research and education). Treatment outcome is postulated as resulting from the interaction of all of these factors. Dean's model seems compatible with Engel's and provides more specificity for therapists.

At a more philosophical level, Ashworth and his colleagues have attempted to outline a framework for understanding patient partici-pation in nursing care (44). Their observations for nursing seem rele-vant to many other health care professionals. These physicians have suggested a synthesis of patient-centered and physician-centered approaches to interviewing that honors the contributions of both par-ties in the partnership (45).

Evidence

Some published research evidence supports selected aspects of these models, although the authors may not have had these models specifi-cally in mind. A major national study on patients' perspectives on their own health care has recently been published involving over 6000 recently hospitalized patients and 2000 care partners (46). As Gerteis and her associates point out, there are two aspects to quality in health care: technical excellence and subjective experience. It is through their subjective experiences that patients define the quality of their health care. Many problems identified by patients have to do with interactions of the patient and health care provider, including not being given infor-mation, getting conflicting information from different health care pro-fessionals, and excluding their families from planning (46).

Ellers (47) noted that family and other significant caregivers ". . . can have a far greater impact on patients' experience of illness, and on their long-term health and happiness, than any health care professional."

One person's illness often affects many peoples' lives, yet the evidence suggests that patients often perceive the exclusion of these people from decision-making process and the information loop (47–49). "Patients are usually satisfied with the technical quality of care they receive. But somewhere in the process, their individuality is lost sight of; their personal and subjective needs remain unmet" (50).

Many researchers have clearly documented the power of the patients' perceptions to influence their interactions with their health care professional and the quality of their therapeutic outcomes (51). Roberson found that health care professionals and patients often had very different definitions of compliance and had differing treatment goals in mind; the patients' definition included feelings of good health and routines that fit their life-styles and personal priorities. Yet Roberson noted that patients were seldom asked about their perspectives on such issues (52).

Sluijs and her colleagues published a correlational study of the sources of patient nonadherence to exercise recommendations in physical therapy (53). Their materials included responses from 222 therapists, 1837 taped therapy sessions, and 1681 patient questionnaires. Their data supported the idea of three primary factors in patient noncompliance: perceived and encountered barriers such as lack of time or pain, lack of positive feedback, and perceived degree of helplessness.

Each of these findings could, at least potentially, be influenced by patient-therapist interaction. DiMatteo and DiNicola also listed three primary causes of noncompliance: intrapsychic factors such as depression, environmental factors such as a busy work schedule, and the practitioner-patient relationship (54). Physicians are frustrated when their patients do not adhere to medical regimens yet often do not know what to do about it. Delbanco had a number of suggestions for improving this situation (55). The frustration that exists between the American public and the health care system and its providers is at a critical level and the root of the problem is personal (56). The medical system has lost touch with its constituency, patients, and essential mission of meeting the needs of patients. Many of the suggestions for improvement involve better communication between the patient and the provider.

In an interesting experiment, Greenfield and his colleagues taught patients how to read their medical record, ask questions, and discuss their care with their physicians before an office visit (57). A control group received a standard patient education program on their disease. About 2 months later, the experimental group reported significantly fewer limitations on their activities, expressed a preference for a greater role in decision-making concerning their care, and were more satisfied with their care than the control group. The experimental group was twice as effective as the controls in obtaining information from their provider. Malzer studied the assessment of patient independence after discharge from a physical rehabilitation unit; assessments were made by rehabilitation nurses, occupational therapists, physical therapists, and the patients (58). No statistically significant correlations were found among the various ratings, suggesting to the author a need for better communications among those involved.

The evidence is much more complex than what one might presume based on the literature reviewed thus far. Two studies using grounded theory did in-depth interviews of patients (59,60). The first study revealed that some patients participate in planning their care because they think that is what the *nurse* wants them to do, rather than what *they* want to do. The researchers concluded that promoting individualized care and active patient involvement are not necessarily the same. The second nursing study concluded that the desire of patients to be involved in decision-making depended on several factors; they were less likely to want to be actively involved the more ill they felt, the more technical they thought the problem was, and the less they trusted their own capabilities. In another study of 210 patients with hypertension and their physicians, only 41% wanted more information than they were given (61). The physicians underestimated their patients' desire for information and overestimated their desire for involvement in decision-making.

Many patients who preferred not to be involved in initial decision-making wanted to be involved in ongoing evaluation of outcomes. We found some evidence suggesting that patients were less interested in decision-making while critically ill, but developed an interest in participation as their problems began to be resolved (62). In a subsequent study, 68% of our subjects said they would have liked more involvement in setting their treatment goals in physical therapy and 47% said they would have liked more involvement in treatment choices. Although these subjects were not asked about adherence, it is not unreasonable to see a connection between these data and adherence (63).

Chiou and Burnett studied the values that patients and their physical and occupational therapists attached to various activities of daily living (ADL) (64). As groups, patients and therapists ranked the ADL similarly; however, only one of the 29 patient-therapist pairs gave significantly similar opinions concerning the value of each ADL for that particular patient, which suggests that these patients and their therapists were working toward different goals.

Carpenter reported a qualitative study of 10 patients with spinal cord injury (24). Although acknowledging the contributions of rehabilitation personnel in the technical aspects of learning to live with their impairments, the subjects emphasized recovery of self, redefining disability, and establishing a new identity as more significant aspects of their learning to live with their disability. As a result of her findings, Carpenter recommended a more client-centered approach to rehabilitation practice.

Brody and his colleagues studied the relationships among patients' perceptions of their roles during a visit to their physicians, their subsequent attitudes about their illness and treatment, and their perception of their improvement (65). Forty-seven percent reported playing an active role during the visit; this group subsequently reported significantly less discomfort and greater improvement in their general health 1 week later. The more active participants also reported a greater sense of control over their illness and more satisfaction with their physicians 1 day after the visit. In one series of semistructured interviews designed to elicit patients' perceptions of their involvement in planning their physical therapy program, patient participation in evaluating outcomes received the strongest support in these patients' experience, participation in the assessment of what helped them received somewhat less support, and patient involvement in goal-setting received the weakest support from the data.

In a related study with patients in occupational therapy, more support was found for patient involvement in goal setting and less support for their involvement in outcomes assessment (66). Occupational therapists also miss many opportunities to involve patients in their own program planning (67). Many patients express a desire for more involvement in their health care than what they actually experienced, but not all; what distinguishes those who want more involvement from those who do not is not immediately obvious. It is clear that the opportunities should be available for participation in all aspects of the planning process to enable the patient-professional interaction to optimize the degree of participation appropriate for each individual.

Patient follow-through in response to recommendations of health care professionals is improved when the expectations of patients regarding their treatment are met, which is more likely to occur when there is agreement between the expectations of the patient and the therapist. Effective communication skills, including attentive listening and the use of clear understandable language, will improve the effectiveness of the therapist and lead to increased patient satisfaction and improved follow-through or adherence (68). Martin and Tubbert demonstrated an increase in patient follow-through in an exercise program when the person was involved in goal setting during program planning (69).

WHAT ARE THE GOALS?

The assumptions that underlie the procedures to be described in this book are that the goals that arise from the persons involved are more likely to receive the investment of energy that will bring them to fruition. It is the client alone who can ultimately determine whether a goal is worth the effort; as much as is consistent with clarity, the goals should be stated in the patient's own language. Once the goals are stated the client can in turn participate in the ongoing process of evaluation of outcomes and of the activities used to achieve such outcomes. Patient participation in planning can thus underlie the entire therapeutic process, making it more effective and more efficient.

In an important sense, the process being described is based also on recognition of the values of self-determination and the worth of the individual. The goal is to integrate the professional's competence in interpreting signs and symptoms and in the technical application of treatments, while emphasizing that planning and evaluative skills must be shared with the client. It is the client who must ultimately be prepared to deal with the problems and to do so not only in the short-term but, in many instances, throughout the rest of his or her life. Patient participation in planning can be the context for learning an important skill for the future, along with the more traditional skills, such as ADL and mobility, learned in rehabilitation settings.

The goal of this book is integral to the overall goal of therapy and of therapy schools that state that the student/clinician will be able to solve problems effectively. It is assumed that clinical problem-solving is both internal and interactive. The internal aspect is concerned with the process that goes on in the health professional's head as he or she deals with the data provided in the clinical interview, in history taking, and in evaluation. From all these sources the clinician must determine both the impairments and the disabilities to develop an appropriate treatment plan including goals, means, and time line. Goals, means, and time line comprise a therapeutic plan, as will be discussed in subsequent chapters.

The determination of the patient's disabilities and the functional consequences of impairment involve an interactive problem-solving process. The interactive part of the process involves the patient from the start in the definition of the problem and decisions about goals. Eventually, the therapist also involves the patients in the evaluation of outcomes and the efficacy of treatments and thus enables participation in all aspects of a plan. It is the interactive aspect of clinical problem-solving that this book describes and it is this interactive aspect where communication skills are essential.

It is also important to say what this book does not do. It is not a complete textbook on communication with patients in the therapeutic setting. Although it may be considered in the context of psychosocial aspects of clinical practice, it is not a primer in patient counseling. It also does not attempt to be a textbook on clinical problem-solving in occupational and physical therapy in all its aspects. This book is specifically one that describes a method for involving patients in self-directed management of those aspects of their lives affected by their disabilities. In so doing, it is likely that therapists will be dealing with an area of the patient's life that is crucial to the person's needs.

In their area of professional competence both physical and occupational therapists will increase their ability to enable persons with disabilities to enhance their function and sense of self-worth.

Sluijs and her colleagues analyzed audiotapes of physical therapy treatment sessions of 1837 patients and concluded that therapists differ widely in their emphasis on patient education (70). Yet an earlier review of literature indicated that patient education was important to practitioner-patient relationships and patient adherence to medical advice (71).

One major objective of education is to influence the attitudes of students toward their future patients. An **attitude** is a learned capability that amplifies the student's positive or negative reaction toward some situation, person, or thing. The strength of an attitude is indicated by the frequency with which one *chooses* that item in a variety of circumstances. Instruction can be effective in modifying attitudes and a part of the method includes presenting models and establishing the appeal and credibility of these models; acquiring particular attitudes may presuppose the learning of specific information (72). Specified knowledge, skills, and values are needed for effective practitioner-patient relationships. They include self-awareness, incorporating patient experience of health and illness, developing and maintaining caring relationships, and effective communication.

Many professionals now prefer a model of illness that includes psychosocial elements and incorporates the patient into the decision-making process. Evidence indicates that patient adherence is enhanced if the patients are involved in decision-making about their own care. Learning about models of care and related information is recommended as a part of the effective education of students.

Therefore, the overall objective of this book is that the student/clinician will be able to plan a therapeutic regimen with a client and maintain patient participation throughout the therapeutic process, including ongoing evaluation of outcomes and means.

Enabling objectives include:

1. Determining the major problems that bring the patient to therapy, with maximal patient input.

2. Generating a specific goal statement in an area relevant to the patient's major problems, with patient participation to the maximal extent possible.

3. Evaluating the goals initially set with maximum patient participation.

4. Revising goals and the time by which goals will be accomplished with maximum patient participation.

5. Specifying the treatment procedures and equipment needs with maximum patient participation.

APPLICATION TO ONESELF I

Another important part of effective education is application to oneself. Starting with this chapter and further detailed in the following chapters, you will be asked to apply the process described in this book to your own problems in education or in clinical practice. You are asked to function in planning your own educational program as an analogy for the type of activity you will then carry out with your clients.

Having experienced the planning process personally, you are then led to experiment with the process in interviews with others. As you grow in the use of this approach, the number of questions addressed in the planning process becomes greater. The skills sought are to be able to define your own answers to a series of planning questions, then to enable patients to do the same. This is done in stages that can be reflected in components of a course that will extend over time and be integrated with a concomitant increase in your clinical skills and experience.

What Are My Concerns?

The exercise presented in Table 1-1 marks the beginning of such participation. The question about concerns/problems marks the beginning of the planning process. Table 1-2 illustrates the application of

Table 1-1 by a reader to herself. Table 1-3 is an example of a list of concerns generated by a group of practicing therapists. If you have difficulty in describing your own concerns, you may select from those listed by others.

Table 1-1.

1. **What are my concerns about involving patients in the planning of their treatment?** List at least 3, and indicate which one you consider to be the most important by placing an asterisk next to it.

   A.

   B.

   C.

Table 1-2.

1. **What are my concerns about involving patients in the planning of their treatment?** List at least 3, and indicate which one you consider to be the most important by placing an asterisk next to it.

   A. Patients with cognitive deficits.

   B. Patient unable to comprehend the questions asked.

   C. Goals that are too general.*

Table 1-3. (Group)

1. **What are your concerns about involving patients in the planning of their treatment?**

   A. Different levels of participation: e.g., patients who are depressed, want to be left alone; patients who use denial of any problem; unmotivated patients; different levels of cognitive function; problems in developing trust in a short time; the limits of patient versus professional responsibility.

   B. Goals not in agreement: e.g., problems in communication; setting unrealistic goals; patient's goals not in agreement with those of professional; rapidly changing goals.

   C. Follow-through of goals: e.g., carry over postdischarge, families unable to carry out goals due to lack of understanding; parents able to follow through as therapists interfering with the parental role.

Chapter 2

The Planning Process

THE GOALS OF THE CHAPTER

THE PLANNING QUESTIONS
What Are the Problems?
What Are the Goals?
What Are the Outcomes?
What May Have Helped?

PLANNING FOR ONESELF II
What Are My Goals?

THE GOALS OF THE CHAPTER

Chapter 1 explored the problems we now face in providing services to persons with disabilities. This chapter describes the procedures by which you can alleviate these problems. The procedures are those of a specified planning process in which certain questions are asked. By the end of this chapter, you should be able to

21

understand the questions, their import, and the steps used in answering them.

THE PLANNING QUESTIONS

The process of rehabilitation treatment is an ongoing planning/evaluation system as described in Figure 2-1. After an initial assessment, a plan is made and implemented with evaluation integral to such implementation; a new plan is made when indicated. This cyclical process can be repeated until the problem has been solved (73).

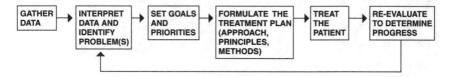

Figure 2-1.   Treatment planning process. (From Trombly CA. *Occupational Therapy for Physical Dysfunction.* 2nd ed. Baltimore: Williams & Wilkins; 1983, with permission.)

Table 2-1 lists the questions to be addressed, each of which is answered in several steps. These steps of exploration, selection, and specification are illustrated with respect to each of the questions.

Table 2-1. The Planning Questions

1. What problems exist? What problems bring you to therapy?
2. What are the goals?
3. What outcomes have been achieved?
4. What has succeeded in producing such outcomes?

What Are the Problems?

The steps leading to the development of a treatment plan start with defining the problem(s). Only after problems have been identified can goals be set as one of the important parts of the total treatment plan. That treatment plan will also contain the methods to be used and the time line.

In making an initial assessment, it is common practice to ask the patient some version of the question "What brings you to therapy?". It is often identified in interview forms as "Chief Complaint." Although such information is sought from the patient and is frequently expressed in the patient's own words, the "actual" problem is usually defined otherwise. The professional defines the problem by some sort of "objective" test or assessment tool that is therefore normally considered more valid as a basis for planning treatment.

The basis for defining the problem is crucial to the entire process. It is important to distinguish between different levels of thinking about human performance. Napier (20) described three different levels. The first is the structural performance at the level of individual anatomic components, such as the knee joint. The second level is the interaction of the various structural components to perform an action such as walking. At the third or behavioral level, the functional components are further combined to act in the context of a setting such as one's work. Here an example might be the ability to get around to deliver the mail if that is one's job.

It is helpful to make the distinction between impairments and disabilities as defined by the World Health Organization (74). When assessing a patient by means of a neurologic examination, muscle testing, joint range of motion, or grip strength, the degree of impairment is being defined. The clinician is assessing, for example, the weakness of the knee extensors as a deviation from the normal of that person or for persons in general. The therapist is assessing at the level of structure. The purpose of rehabilitation is frequently not to deal with the underlying impairments, which may remain stable. Paraplegia after a spinal cord injury or hemiparesis after a stroke or head injury may not be subject to change by the therapist. Along with the prevention of further impairment, the purpose of rehabilitation is to deal with the reorganization of the patient (in respect to skills and attitudes) so that the person can better deal with the functional consequences of such impairments. The purpose is to reduce the degree of disability. It is the definition of these disabilities that requires input from the clients; these functional consequences must be defined in terms of the person who is experiencing them.

For example, as a result of paraplegia, the patient may have difficulty getting around. He or she may not be able to get out of bed or maneuver a wheelchair. Even more specifically, as a result of the weakness of the knee extensors, the individual cannot stand to transfer from the bed to a chair. A survivor of a stroke with a paralyzed upper extremity cannot cut meat or tie a shoe. It is the loss of mobility, the inability to transfer, or the inability to grasp a utensil or to pinch a shoelace that is the disability. Furthermore, it is the person with the problem (or family) who can best define what is often an individualistic effect of the impairments. It is even more necessary to select from the various impairments those that are actually disabling to that person. Contrary to what is usually done, it is the subjective problem that is to be the basis for an effective treatment plan.

The following example comes from an interview with a woman who had developed a left hemiplegia after an occlusion of one of the blood vessels of the brain:

THERAPIST: What are your problems?

PATIENT: My left side is weak.

THERAPIST: What problems does your weakness on your left side cause you?

PATIENT: I have trouble going up and down steps.

THERAPIST: What sort of trouble do you have going up and down steps?

PATIENT: I'm afraid I will lose my balance on my steep front steps.

Only the person can best determine, in the context of her own life setting, the specific aspects that are disabling about the impairment in her left side. Still another person with the same impairment may have a quite different life setting, with different consequences. Similarly, when one considers the number of potential areas of disability for the person with left-sided weakness exemplified by this lady (such as mobility, dressing, transfers), all may be relevant to the person's goals. Some, however, may be of a higher priority in light of personal characteristics such as goals and resources. For example, it may be less important for a person to take the time to learn to dress herself given the severity of her impairments. She may plan to have an attendant help with that activity if necessary to be able to get to work on time.

Still another aspect has been achieved by addressing the question as to the problem in this way. The professional must help the patient move as this patient did from defining the problem in terms of impairment of her left side to the consequent functional disability. It is for this reason that the professional must be clear about the distinction to help the patient make this transition to consider the functional aspects. Although the weakness of the left side may be unchangeable, the clinician can enable the person to get in and out of her house if that is the problem. It may, however, be necessary to modify the environment by use of an outside elevator, or more likely, by use of alternative ways of getting into the house. This looking for alternative ways to accomplish goals is the work of rehabilitation. The first step, however, is to define the problem in these more functional terms.

In establishing as clearly as possible the problem at any one time, it is useful to explore the question at least three times. In this step of exploration, it is important to avoid making judgments. During the next step of selection, one will judge in some way with the patient what might be the highest priority problem or the clearest statement of the problem. Threefold exploration is a useful minimum but may not always be sufficient to define the problem adequately. The ongoing quality of the therapist-client relationship permits re-exploration at any time. One may explore "in depth," as with the woman described earlier with left-sided weakness. The question was asked in a successive way by incorporating the answer previously given.

Alternatively, one may explore "in breadth," as in the following example:

THERAPIST: What problems do you have?
PATIENT: I have a tingling in my left side.
THERAPIST: Is there anything else that troubles you?
PATIENT: I have trouble using my left ankle.
THERAPIST: Is there anything else?
PATIENT: I can't move my toes.
THERAPIST: What bothers you the most?
PATIENT: It's hard for me to walk.

In this case, the threefold exploration step did not identify a clear statement. It was possible to define a relatively clear statement describing a problem at a functional level in the next selection step. It is this last statement that can become the basis for generating a goal statement. After exploring these several alternatives and only then making a selection, the likelihood is greater that the eventual goal will actually be relevant to the patient's needs.

In this next example of an interview with a person with paraplegia due to a spinal cord injury, three problems were explored. As is frequently the case, it is the third statement that was the major concern. In this instance, the patient explored for himself and made a selection himself.

THERAPIST: What problems are you having due to your spinal cord injury?
PATIENT: I don't know. Let me think. I am not bothered by using a wheelchair to get around. I can keep up with people.

> Things are going OK with my wife. This may sound
> crazy to you. What really bothers me is that I used to
> be a tall person. Now that I am sitting in a wheelchair,
> I can't reach what I used to be able to reach. I am now
> a short person. That really bothers me.

The time spent initially in the process of exploring a problem leading to its definition is generally well spent. In a recent interview, a person with amputations of both legs of many years' duration was asked
about her concerns now that she had a new second set of prostheses.
In the process of the threefold exploration of the question regarding her
concerns, she described for her therapist for the first time what she later
said had troubled her for the past 10 years with her old prostheses. She
stated that she had always been concerned about injuring herself if she
fell. What bothered her even more was that she lived alone and had
never learned how to get herself up again after falling. She was afraid
she would not be able to get help. Earlier, she had not had the chance
nor did she feel she had the right to express what she felt she needed.
At this time, on the basis of her exploration, she established as one of
her priorities the goal of learning how to get herself up off the floor and
how to minimize her injuries if she fell.

In the examples thus far, we have illustrated asking the patient to
simply select the most important concern or problem from those elicited
during exploration. The therapist may go about the process of selection
in a number of different ways. There are different bases for attaching
priorities. Therapists identified several different reasons that they can
offer patients to help them make a selection. One could select on the
basis of the problem most frequently encountered, the severity of the
problem, the one that could be the most difficult to overcome, or even
the one that would be the easiest to overcome.

More complex methods of prioritizing could also be used. One
could ask patients to rank in order that which they consider first, second, and third. Still another approach is to weigh the several options by
assigning a sharing of value to each pair. This technique permits a later
rough approximation of allocation of resources, such as time, to each
of the priorities. For example, if there are three concerns, one can compare the assignment of weights within each pair such as A and B, then
A and C, then B and C. If a total of 3 points is assigned, one could
assign 3 points to A and none to B; or 2 to A and 1 to B, and so forth,
for a total of 9 points. The following example was elicited by an occupational therapist working with a patient:

THERAPIST: What problems bring you to therapy?
PATIENT: A. I can't drive to get around.
            B. I don't have many outside interests.
            C. I can't propel my wheelchair very far.
THERAPIST: How important to you are each of these problems?
            Share 3 points between each of paired items.
            A. 3 2 (5)
            B. 0 1 (1)
            C. 1 2 (3)

With this method, no item is discarded. Yet the process of sharing weights provides some greater clarification of the proper allocation of resources to the resolution of the problems identified during the exploration step. One could allocate 5/9 of the resources such as time to item A; 1/9 to item B; and 3/9 to item C.

Now that one has explored the concerns and made some judgment as to priorities in the selection step, the next step is to specify the problem. For example, the statement "my shoulder hurts" merely answers the question about what the problem may be. A more specific statement would be "my shoulder hurts at night so that I can't sleep." Such a statement answers not only what (pain in the shoulder) but also when (at night) and how much (so that I can't sleep). It is generally useful to specify the chief complaint generated during the selection step to the extent that it meets a 3-point criterion. That criterion could be met by answering not only "What?" but also either "When?" or "Where?" in terms of the setting, and "How much?" or "How long?" or some other measure addressing the degree. The issue of the methods for carrying out the specification step are addressed in greater detail in relation to the next question in the planning process dealing with the identification of a goal.

The process of defining a problem is a crucial first step in designing a treatment plan. For some, it is quite difficult to even address this question. The wording of the question can vary depending on the context. Some therapists have found using the word "concerns" to be unclear. Synonyms can be used such as "worries," "problems," or "troubles." In some situations, the word "questions" can be used. Some may deny that a problem exists. The very process of thinking about one's problems may be overpowering. By one's willingness to state what one is worried about, a certain distance occurs in relation to the problem. In relation to one's worries, the client can be active or passive. The person can be their victim as in "it worries me," or try to master them as in "I am worried about something." The message being sent by asking this question is that one can begin to look at one's problems and that they can be defined in functional terms.

The answers will vary with the person's own type and degree of impairment. The answers will also vary with the persons' individualistic setting, resources, and goals. It is important also to recognize that the problem statement made by the client may change over time as thoughts become clearer, as problems are solved and new problems appear, and as the client feels more trust in the person who is asking. The ability to answer this or any other of the questions also depends on the skill of patients in verbalizing what they are thinking or feeling. It is the task of the professional to enable patients to answer this question as freely and as fully as possible, recognizing the probability of limited success at any one time.

What Are the Goals?

The aim is to generate a "specific" goal statement in an area relevant to the patient's main concern. We have looked at the process of identifying the major concern. Once the problem has been adequately identified and defined, the next step in the planning process is to establish goals that, when accomplished, would indicate that the problem has been alleviated. The phrasing of this question can vary. You can ask in a straightforward way: "What are your goals for therapy?" or "What do you hope to accomplish in therapy?" or "What do you expect to get out of therapy?". Alternatively, you can ask: "What would make you think (or feel) that things are going better?" The goal statement describes an outcome, the results being sought.

Just as with the question as to problem, a message is being sent when this question is asked. The message is that a potential for change exists and that change might be for the better. The willingness of patients to address this question depends on a sense that they can look to a better future. Addressing this question may be very difficult for those who have just had a severe loss in their ability to function or to care for their own most basic needs, such as after a stroke or spinal cord injury. The ability to speak to this question might therefore develop only on the basis of experience with results having been accomplished as part of an ongoing planning process.

The goal would ordinarily derive from the main concern. For example, if the main concern was the inability to dress oneself, then one possible goal could be "to be able to put on a shirt." One concern listed in the previous section was "Pain in the left shoulder at night so that I can't sleep." Evidence that the problem is being solved relating to the expressed concern can vary depending on the person who is experiencing the pain. One such goal statement could be "have the pain go away." Another could be "not have the pain interfere with my sleep, be able to get my usual 8 hours of sleep." Still another even more functional goal could be "feel well rested in the morning when I have to go to work." The treatment portion of the plan would vary somewhat depending on the goal statement eventually identified.

Another person with a recent spinal cord injury can illustrate the value of the process of addressing the question of goal in relation to the stated concern. He was concerned about the pain in the legs he was experiencing below the level of injury. He identified his major concern to be knowing what the pain meant. His goal was to find out whether the leg pain meant that something was seriously wrong. He met his goal when he was reassured that pain below the level of injury in persons with spinal cord injury did not necessarily signify that something serious was happening, as it may have before the injury. The therapist cannot presuppose what a person's goal may be. The therapist cannot assume that because the client has pain the goal will always be the reduction of the pain. It is necessary to ask about the person's goals.

A minimum of three possible goals are explored before one is selected as the highest priority, which is then specified. The exploration step is useful in dealing with the need to define the problem in functional terms. The transition between the normal patient focus on the impairments to that of the functional consequences or disabilities may not as yet have been fully accomplished. As an example, one woman stated her concern: "I can't use my left arm." Her first goal statement thus dealt with regaining strength in her affected arm. In exploring other possible goals she was able eventually to identify a functional goal that could be accomplished more readily. The sequence of further exploration went as follows:

THERAPIST: Everyone is different. The trouble with your hand can affect you and your life differently from another person. What sorts of things would you like to be able to do that would make you feel that you are doing better?
PATIENT: I'd like to be able to do more to take care of my children.
THERAPIST: What sorts of things would make you feel that you are doing something for your children?
PATIENT: I guess I could cook for them.

The exploration step can serve still another purpose. One further value is that the exploration can reduce the likelihood that the goals will be unrealistic. One young man with a recent spinal cord injury initially stated his goal "to be like I was before my injury." When asked whether he had any other goals, his next statement was "to be an athlete the way I was before." When asked once again in a nonjudgmental exploration step, his next statement was "to understand the extent of my injuries and how they affect my future." Such exploration increases the possibility of some goals that can be shared by both the therapist and the client. Similarly, the patient may initially mention a goal that may require a much longer term commitment than is usually available in the service setting. It is possible to ask the patient to consider some short-term goals in this exploration step. The therapist may phrase the question as follows: "What might be a first step in meeting your goal?" It is generally possible for at least one short-term goal to arise that meets the joint needs of both the therapist and the client.

It is highly important to enable the patient to keep what may be to another "an impossible dream" while still defining some intermediate goals that would indicate progress. For example, in the case of the person with brain injury whose ultimate goal might be to walk again, an intermediate goal compatible with walking could be to be able to stand or maintain one's balance while sitting. It is helpful to maintain the connection between the short-term goal and the ultimate one. It is often quite surprising to the therapist how much can be accomplished by people with disabilities with the will to do so. It is not necessary to spend one's energy to deprive people of their long-term goals that may seem unrealistic to the therapist. If one goes about setting short-term goals and reviewing outcomes in an ongoing process, the realities of the rate of progress can clarify what can be accomplished for both the client and the professionals.

Another source of conflict in the expectations between the therapist and patient lies in the patient's unwillingness to consider short-term intermediate goals based on the sense that time alone will heal. Many have the mistaken belief that improvement will occur spontaneously over some months and only then do they see the need to commit themselves to dealing with whatever disabilities still remain. There are undoubtedly opportunities for recovery in the early weeks or months after injury. This is particularly true for persons with stroke and other forms of brain injury. This is far less true for persons with spinal cord injury if the injury is "complete." What can happen in the meantime is worsening of the degree of underlying impairment such as the formation of contractures and other illness in the urinary tract and skin due to lack of care. The best antidote to the sense of hopelessness and passivity is the effort to set even low-level goals that can provide the basis for the experience that progress does occur.

It is important at this juncture to distinguish between goals and means. The goal statement relates to the outcomes, the results, the "ends" of the therapeutic activities. Persons enter into rehabilitation because they have lost some of the ways (means) by which they have ordinarily performed their life activities. It may not always be possible for them to regain those ways. What is generally far more likely is that they can regain the functional results that those now lost means enabled them to achieve. For example, although walking may be preferred, it may no longer be possible to use walking to get around in the same way as before. It will still be possible to get around if that was what walking accomplished for the person. However, walking was generally not the only method the client had for getting around in the past. For example, the automobile and even the horse in some rural settings were likely modes of getting around before the injury. It is often now necessary to use alternative methods or means to accomplish the goal of mobility. The goals can remain the same to a great degree. What frequently must change are the means. This distinction must be clear to the professional to enable the patient to bridge this gap and consider alternative ways of doing things that may be ultimately acceptable.

In the case of the woman with the weak left hand, she naturally focused first on the loss of strength in that hand. It was important to enable her to consider that the strong hand was but a means to the end of caring for her children. Although making her task more difficult than before, the weakness need not preclude her from accomplishing one of her goals. She was able to look toward a functional goal by being essentially asked the question "Why?" in relation to her left arm. "Why does your weakness in your left arm trouble you?" "What would you be trying to accomplish with your arm if it were stronger?" She eventually set a goal of making breakfast for her children, which was both short-term and still compatible with her overall goal of caring for her children.

The change in focus toward caring for her children rather than the left arm itself enabled her to consider alternative ways of doing things. Goals such as increased range of motion and increased strength are measurable and desirable but may be only means to the functional goals that are the ultimate basis for judgment of outcome. The threefold exploration step is an opportunity to aid this major change in thinking.

Just as the chief complaint could be selected, prioritized, or determined by a weighting system, so too the primary or first-order goal statement can be derived by any of those procedures. It is this first-order or short-term goal that can be specified.

The specification step is particularly useful in relation to the goal statement because it will provide the basis for answering the next question as to outcome in the ongoing planning process. The statement of the goal must be specific to be measurable. If it is measurable, it will be easier to demonstrate its achievement. Thus far, in the exploratory and selection steps, the goal statement had merely to answer the question as to "What?". To meet the criterion of "specificity," it is also necessary to answer the questions of "Where?" or "When?" in dealing with the setting in which the goal is to be accomplished. The setting in time in which the outcome is to be demonstrated can be an interview, the therapy session, and so forth. (The time line, the duration of the time before the goal is to reached, is a separate item in the total plan.) The third question to be answered to meet the criteria for specificity is some measure as to degree such as "How much?" or "How far?" or "How well?".

Examples of specific goal statements are:

What? Generate a goal statement

When? In an interview

How well? To meet the 3-point criterion

What? Walk

How far? For 5 feet

Where? Between parallel bars

When? During the therapy session

What? Turn over from side to side

Where? In the hospital bed

How often? Every 3 hours

What Are the Outcomes?

The initial specification of the goal statement permits evaluation of outcomes to occur in this first recycling of the planning process. One can recall that therapy or rehabilitation can be seen as a recurrent planning cycle. The process includes the making of a plan consisting of a goal statement, a time for review, and a set of treatments or means by which the goal is to be reached. In this review step, the first new question relates to the evaluation of the goal. There will also be an opportunity to review the treatments carried out. Following these questions, the initial plan can be revised.

One concern of therapists is the maintenance of commitment by patients with chronic impairments to perform what may be strenuous activities, particularly when such activities need to go on over a rather long time. To a lesser extent, commitment may also be a problem for those with short-term difficulties. What has thus far been accomplished in setting an initial goal is but a necessary first step in dealing with this problem. The need to maintain enthusiasm is not limited to the patient but also applies to staff to prevent "burnout." One must see results, and those results must somehow be connected to what was being sought. The need for documentation of results is also required by third-party payers and accreditation agencies.

It is important to review the goals initially established and to relate this new question to the work done before. The same three steps are used for answering this question as the previous ones. In the exploration step, the threefold description of outcomes can re-enforce the sense that some results did occur. As one therapist expressed it, "The patient hearing himself describe some positive outcomes helps the person to feel better about what has been happening. It helps the patient to keep putting out the effort necessary." Because that is the aim, the exploration of at least three aspects of any outcome or three different outcomes can contribute to a sense of hope that progress will continue to occur.

The exploration step may require consideration of intermediate or even shorter term goals than originally set. One may find that the original set was not met in its entirety. One may find that many more small incremental steps are necessary. There is thus another opportunity to set new goals with greater awareness on the part of the therapist and the patient of the rate with which progress can come. It is important, however, to connect the progress that did occur, albeit partial, to the goal that was originally set. Alternatively, larger or unanticipated accomplishments may have occurred.

The subsequent selection step can be based on either of the techniques for selection illustrated in relation to the questions about concerns and goals. One may determine the result about which the person feels the best or remembers best. The value of making a selection lies in focusing the patient on a scene that can then more readily relived. A major objective of this outcome question is to enable the person to savor and potentially take hope from the accomplishments, rather than report a failure to do so. It is sometimes preferable to review the present status of the patient rather than merely review whether the goal in its entirety was accomplished or not. Attention to the actual newly achieved status can obviate the need to focus on failure if the initial goal was not fully met.

The specification of the selected outcome should describe not only "What?" had been accomplished but also "When?" and "Where?". Answering both these questions about the setting can aid in visualizing the experience. By recalling that scene, the patient can more readily relive and savor it. Criteria of specificity would also include some measure of degree such as "How far?" or "How much?". An example of a specific statement might be "I just now walked 5 feet in my room." In the context of reviewing the scene, the person may then be better able to consider the next question reviewing the actions that may have contributed to the outcome.

What May Have Helped to Achieve the Results?

The characteristics of a plan include not only a goal but also the means by which that goal is to be achieved and a time line for the review to be performed. The additional question as to the means can now be asked after having described some of the outcomes achieved. Evocation of the scene in terms of where and when it occurred can provide the context for defining the actions taken that may have been helpful. One is seeking to determine the efficacy of the procedures. For an activity to be efficacious, it must be viewed as having the power to produce the desired effect. Not only must there be the desired effect, but a relationship must be established between the action(s) taken and the outcome of those actions.

Just as with the previous questions, the asking of this new question conveys a possible message to change the person's perceptions. What should be conveyed is that what has occurred is in some way related to actions that were taken, particularly actions taken by the patient. Once again, this may require a major change in thinking. Some have great difficulty in making that connection. For example, one man with problems in his speech due to disease affecting his motor system noted that his speech could vary from day to day or at times during the course of the day. He spoke spontaneously about the existence of this problem. He was also able to monitor his performance. He was willing to address the question as to outcome. However, he was not willing to consider the question as to what may be useful to affect the results he witnessed. For example, he would not consider that it was helpful to take a breath at the start of a sentence so that he would not run out of breath or use any of the other techniques recommended by his speech therapist.

A major effect of impairment has been the loss of control of one's body with serious implications for a loss of a sense of control in one's life. The development of a sense of personal contribution to the achievement of positive outcomes can be a crucial component to the ultimate goal of regaining a sense of control over one's life. The sense that the actions leading to success have been taken by the patient rather than some outside agent is an important aspect of the development of a sense of efficacy of the person involved. It is this sense of personal efficacy in problem-solving that is an aim along with a greater awareness of some of the ways such outcomes were achieved.

The exploration step, once again threefold, is designed to increase the patient's awareness that options exist and an awareness of what those options are. In many instances, the person becomes a patient and enters into rehabilitation after having lost some of the ways by which he or she ordinarily performed activities significant to everyday life. An important part of the rehabilitative process is recognition of alternative ways of doing things, of adapting or compensating. These new ways are by their very nature "abnormal" in that they are usually different from the ways the person previously accomplished these same daily goals. By being new and different, at least at the start, they are also frequently more difficult. It is important in the interaction between the patient and the therapist that every opportunity be used to increase the sense that activities can be accomplished in more than one way. If only two ways are perceived, a sense of limited choice will still exist. Describing at least three answers to the question can create a sense of freedom, of options.

The subsequent selection step can be based once again on any of the techniques used in dealing with the other questions in the planning process. The basis for making a selection may relate to the actions that seemed to work the best or that are the clearest in one's mind. Another basis for selection can relate to the important issue of the source of the actions that were helpful. Emphasis can be on those actions performed mainly by the client or the particular contribution that the person with the disability made to the actions that were effective. For example, it is common for the person to attribute the results to the use of medication as though it is an agent beyond control. Yet it is the patient's use of the medication in the proper dosage and in relation to some schedule that permits the drug to be effective. It is that set of actions taken by the patient that can be emphasized. Another example of the use of the exploration step can be when the initial answer to the question as to what may have worked is "hot packs." The possible contributions by the patient may have been "heating the hot packs to the proper temperature, putting them on the prescribed place on the body, and making sure that they were on for the whole time." If several ideas are presented during the exploration step, the selection can be the one the patient perceives to have contributed the most.

For example, one man ascribed the improvement in his spasms to "warmer weather," "stretching exercises," and the use of a specific medication. He selected the "stretching exercises" when asked to do so on the basis of what he thought contributed the most. Those exercises can now be specified. It is common in the review process for the patient to describe the activities actually carried out to be different from those initially prescribed. If a nonjudgmental approach has been taken in the exploration of what may have worked, the patient will share what was actually done. The aim is to connect the actions to the results. It is appropriate to revise the actions to be used in the next cycle based on what did seem to be satisfactory. For example, the patient may have varied the frequency or intensity of the exercises, seemingly to good effect. The treatment procedures can be seen to become more to fit to the patient.

The specification of the selected actions should describe the actions to a higher criterion of specificity than used in the answers to the previous questions. A higher degree of specificity is appropriate when describing the technical aspects of either the use of equipment or treatment programs. An exercise program, for example, could be described as "swim 30 minutes three times each week in the health club pool at a peak rate of 130 per minute." Such a statement specifies not only what is to be done and where but also how long, how often, and how fast. One may choose to establish a 5-point criterion of specificity. An example meeting that criterion would be a treatment program such as "apply hot packs (130°F) to the left shoulder three times daily for 30 minutes each time." Still another would be "apply the postoperative arthroplasty splint each day for 22 hours to the extensor surface for the next 2 weeks." This statement includes not only what but where, when, how long, and how often.

Now that there has been a review of both the outcomes and the means by which those outcomes may have been achieved, the initial plan can be revised based on experience. One can now recycle the process by considering the existence of the same or another problem, perhaps a more reasonable goal and a set of procedures that are now modified by experience. Crucial to the effectiveness of this recurrent process is the opportunity to increase the ability of the patient to contribute to the planning. This is the topic of Chapter 3.

PLANNING FOR ONESELF II

What Are My Goals?

In the exercise at the end of Chapter 1, you explored the first question regarding concerns or problems and selected your area of greatest concern. That exercise marked the start of your participation in learning how to use this approach by doing it for yourself. At this point, having reviewed the planning questions, your concerns may be somewhat different from those you originally considered. Your answers may change as you encounter new dimensions of the process of learning to involve patients in a meaningful way in their own program planning. At this time, therefore, you should once again explore your concerns and make a selection. The exploration step can be done in depth if only one problem is identified initially. You can then successively ask the question: "What is troublesome about_____(whatever the expressed concern was)?". You can also explore by listing several problems, asking "What else do I find difficult about learning how to involve patients in their own planning?". You can use Table 2-2 as a format to re-examine your concerns relative to your educational plan. (Please note, circling levels of participation is not done for self-planning.)

Table 2-2. Program Planning Sheet 1 (PPS-1)

Patient _____   Date _____

                                              Therapist _____

PROGRAM PLANNING SHEET 1

1. What are your concerns?
   A.
   B.
   C.

2. What is your greatest concern?
   Check out: _____ agreed _____ confirmed

3. What do you want to see happen? What would make you feel that you are making progress in dealing with your chief concern? What are your goals?
   A.
   B.
   C.

4. What is your specific goal?
   A B C D What?
   A B C D Setting;
   A B C D Degree?

5. Please circle the "lowest" level of participation used in answer to the various portions of the goal statement.
   A = open-ended question: FREE CHOICE
   B = suggestions (3 options): MULTIPLE CHOICE
   C = recommendation (1 option): CONFIRMED CHOICE
   D = recommendation (1 option): FORCED CHOICE
   E = prescription (tell what to do): NO CHOICE

The selection process you use may involve shared weights or simple prioritization. Table 2-3 illustrates the use of shared weights. You can make a selection of the best statement of concern or the most important problem. You may have already specified the problem to the extent of not only what it is but some measure of its severity and setting.

Table 2-3. Example of Use of Weighting to Select Main Concern; Use of Form PPS-1 by Student for Her Own Concerns

Patient _____   Date _____

Therapist _____

PROGRAM PLANNING SHEET 1

1. What are your concerns?

   3   2   = 5   A. I am concerned that I won't be able to use this
                            method with aphasic patients.

   0   1 = 1   B. I'm afraid that I won't remember the questions
                            when I get to the interview.

            1   2 = 3   C. I am concerned that I won't be able to think of
                            multiple-choice options when I need them.

2. What is your greatest concern?

   I am concerned that I won't be able to use this method with
      aphasic patients
   during an interview in clinic
   to the degree that I will be able to elicit patient concerns and goals

   Check out: ___X___ agreed _____ confirmed

3. What would you like to see happen that would make you feel that you
   were making progress with your chief concern?
   A. I will develop a nonverbal communication system with the patient
      (e.g., head nodding).
   B. I will feel comfortable talking to an aphasic person.
   C. I will establish an aphasic patient's concerns and goals.

4. What is your first goal?

   What: I will communicate with an aphasic patient using non-
                verbal communications
   Setting: In an interview in clinic
   Degree: To the degree that I will have a chief complaint and goal
                statement, which the patient agrees to by nodding

---

You may now explore your personal goals in your educational plan for the use of this book by listing three successive steps or three alternative goals (items 3 A-C). Then you would identify the major goal or the one you want to accomplish first. These are your goals in learning the content of this book or course. The final goal statement should be specified as described earlier in this chapter (item 4).

It is important to emphasize the distinction between goals and means. The rehabilitation planning process frequently requires the patient to clarify the distinction between ends (or goals) and means to continue to achieve one's life goals despite the loss of the previously used means. To help patients make this distinction, the therapist must be clear about it. For example, a student/therapist, when asked to state a goal for himself, mentioned "jogging 5 miles a day three times each week." Although this may be a desirable and measurable action, the statement does not define the functional outcome he sought to achieve. It is comparable to many of the goals set by therapists and patients, which are actually activities or means. It was helpful to this student to ask himself why he was going to jog. The outcomes could include weight reduction, increased oxygen efficiency, decreased resting heart rate, increased endurance, and so forth. He could ask the question "Why?" in reference to the outcomes described. He could actually be seeking to increase longevity, reduce the chance of heart disease, and so forth. He could even define the outcomes in terms of why he might be interested in living longer. However, threefold exploration provides a reasonable limit for such activity. Once his goal was identified, he could consider possible alternative means by which his health improvement program could be achieved. Jogging is only one of many means for doing so.

Still another issue that has been difficult for many student/therapists to carry out is the need for personalization of their concerns and goals. Unless able to do so for oneself, it is difficult to help patients to do the same. Personalizing is achieved by the use of personal pronouns. It is a matter of clearly articulating ownership of the concerns and goals with statements such as "I am concerned that _____ " or "I would like to _____." For example, one therapist said: "I am concerned about my ability to help patients set realistic goals." A possible personalized specific goal then could be: "During my next interview, I would like my patient to describe three goals to the degree that they are consistent with what 50% of patients with the same degree of neurologic impairment are able to achieve." Another therapist who had a similar concern did not address her concern when she set a goal as "patient will ambulate independently on the ward for 60 feet." It was a goal for the patient but did not deal with her own concern about her skill in helping patients to set realistic goals.

Tables 2-3 and 2-4 offer examples of how other student/therapists have completed this exercise. The Program Planning Sheet in Table 2-2 is one version of a form used with patients. As we go along, this basic form will change as more questions are added for you to use for yourself and with patients.

Table 2-4. Example of Student Use of Concerns and Goals Sections of the Form

Patient _____   Date _____

                                                  Therapist _____

PROGRAM PLANNING SHEET 1

1. What are your concerns?
   A. I am concerned about integrating this system smoothly into a patient interview.
   B. Will I be able to get the patient to see the difference between goals and means?
   *C. Can I get the patients to "open up" and share his concerns and goals with me?
2. What is your greatest concern?
   Will I be able to get the patient to "open up" and share his concerns and goals with me?

Check out: __*_*__ agreed _____ confirmed

3. What do you want to see happen? What would make you feel that you are making progress? What are your goals?
   A. I will feel comfortable in the interview.
   *B. I will get a clear statement of concerns and goals from the patient.
   C. The patient will talk freely to me.

4. What is your specific goal?
What:	I will complete Form 1
Setting:	During a 20-minute patient interview
Degree:	To the extent that I elicit 3 concerns, a chief concern, 3 goals, and 1 specific goals

Chapter 3

The Patient as Participant

THE GOALS OF THE CHAPTER

One of the overall goals of this book is to enable you to carry out the ongoing planning of a therapeutic regimen with maximal participation by the patient. This requires maintenance of patient participation throughout, including evaluation of goals and means. Chapter 2 described the basic planning questions and how they relate to each other as part of the ongoing planning process. The steps

are used to answer each of the questions. The step of three-fold exploration can provide the data on which the next step of evaluation or
selection occurs. Specification to varying degrees can then be done for
aspects identified in the selection step. This chapter deals with the
degree to which carrying out the several steps and generating the
answers to the planning questions can arise from the patient versus
the professional with the professional being a consultant in planning.
Ultimately, clients can be their own planning consultants with the questions themselves part of their own repertoire to be used as needed.

The aim is for patients to become managers of their own lives,
albeit now in the context of impairment that requires ongoing adaptation. Participation in the rehabilitation planning process, along with the
professional, serves as a training ground for the development of later
independent self-management. The development of such skills goes on
concomitantly with the clinical activities. A participation scale can aid in
the consciousness with which development of such skills occurs. In the
exercise Planning for Oneself III, you should be able to use the format
provided to perform a self-evaluation incorporating the review of your
own initial plan. After reviewing the material in this chapter, in the exercise entitled Application to Patient Care, you can perform the entire
process with another person, including the evaluation of the degree of
participation achieved.

THE PARTICIPATION SCALE

Integral to the use of each of the questions in Chapter 2 is the ultimate
goal of having the answers to the planning questions come from the
client to the maximal degree possible. The two coexisting aims for such
participation to occur are self-knowledge and commitment of energy. It
has been our assumption in dealing with the problem of patient commitment to carrying out the therapy that optimizing participation in the
planning process will increase the degree to which effort will be available for the implementation of any program. Participation can lead to
ownership and thus commitment. The other aim is self-knowledge. One
can increase one's knowledge with both the questions and the answers.
In reference to the answers, verbalization of the answers in the context
of an interested "other" can enable the person to hear better the
answers for oneself. Enhanced self-awareness of one's answers can
bring clarity to what one's problems, goals, and results might be and
what instructions or means might be useful. Ultimately, one can also
increase self-knowledge of the import of the questions regardless of the

content of the answers. One could become more aware that problems do exist, that one can have a sense of direction in dealing with those problems, that one can have a sense of hope when hearing that progress is being made, and that one can have a sense of self-empowerment or self efficacy in bringing about those results.

The objective of maximal participation by the patient does not require any absolute level of participation. Rather it seeks to achieve the highest level of participation consistent with accomplishing the other aims of identifying needs and specifying goals, of describing outcomes and what may work, and carrying out the various steps in doing so. A dialogue is established between the therapist and the patient. Both participants have the right and responsibility to indicate agreement (or disagreement) with the ideas being offered by the other. The exploration step offers an opportunity to reach a common consensus in most instances.

The first question dealing with the identification of the problem clearly depends on such participation. The definition of the individualistic disabilities caused by the impairments will vary with the person and his or her own goals and resources as well as the type and severity of the impairments. Similarly, the goals to be set will vary with the person. The degree to which the therapist can enable clients to participate in stating their goals establishes ownership in the results to be achieved and thus enhanced commitment of energy to their accomplishment. Moreover, clarity regarding the goals provides the basis for ongoing participation in the review of its degree of accomplishment.

Self-awareness of the accomplishments provides the basis for a sense of hope and the data to use for answering the crucial question as to what may have worked to bring about such accomplishments. Our emphasis on patient participation in defining outcomes as well as goals brings the patient into the loop of self-monitoring. This is an essential part of the process. Our experience as well as that of others seeking ongoing implementation of a treatment plan supports the usefulness of inviting such participation. Patient participation in the evaluation and ongoing revision of plans can be expected to maintain a greater degree of participation in an ongoing treatment program.

The ongoing long-term commitment of patients to their care is also enhanced if, during therapy, they learn to be observant of the efforts to meet goals. They can become more nearly the owners of those efforts and methods by modifying them in some way to make them better fit their own circumstances. By participating in the answering of this question of methods or means, clients can now potentially instruct themselves in the actions. The instruction can become internalized and then more automatic. It is in the externalization and focus on the instruction in the context of an interested "other" that the internalization process can be enhanced.

Table 3-1 presents a scale that describes the levels of participation that have been most generally used, listing the order of the degree of involvement in answering the questions. Answering the planning questions reflects the need to perform the various steps of exploration, selection, and specification. The term level is used throughout to refer to the degree of patient participation achieved. For example, the highest level of participation, "free choice," reflects the client originating responses to all three steps in the process with the professional merely

Table 3-1. Levels of Patient Participation

Therapist	Patient	Level
Asks open-ended question	"Free choice" Explores and Selects	A
Asks questions, provides suggestions (3 options)	"Multiple choice" Selects	B
Asks questions, provides an answer (recommendation) and asks for agreement and confirmation	"Confirmed choice" Puts into own words what had been selected	C
Asks question, provides an answer (recommendation) and asks for agreement	"Forced choice" Agrees or (disagrees) with what had been selected	D
Prescribes, does not ask; commands	"No choice" Compliant (or noncompliant)	E

asking the appropriate questions. The patient both explores and selects the answer to "What?" and generates the answers in the further specification questions as to "Where?" and "To what degree?". The next level of participation, "multiple choice," describes the client making the selection step as to "What?" from the alternatives provided by the therapist in the initial step and also selecting from the alternatives provided during the specification process. The next level of participation, "forced choice," describes the selection already made by the professional both for defining "What?" and in the further specification step.

The maximal level of participation is defined as the highest level of participation consistent with meeting the other goals of the interactive planning process. One method for doing so involves starting the interview process with an open-ended question, expecting the patient to act at a "free choice" level. One could then "move down" the scale as necessary only one step at a time to meet the other objectives. Whenever possible, the interviewer should return to the next highest level during the course of the interaction. For example, one could start exploration by asking an open-ended question ("free choice"). It may become necessary to move down the scale to "multiple choice" to achieve threefold exploration. When specifying what had been selected, one should once again attempt to use an open-ended question rather than assume that one must operate at the "multiple choice" level throughout. Similarly, if one had moved down the scale to the "forced choice" level where selection had already been made, it would be desirable to try to move up the scale to "confirmed choice" rather than assume that one must remain at the level of "forced choice" throughout the interaction. The participation score for any particular question can reflect either the highest level of participation achieved or the lowest in carrying out the several steps.

In the forms used, our policy is to record the lowest level of participation achieved as a measure of the commitment that might then be available for implementation. The therapist should seek patient agreement to any change in the level of participation being used and as the person is being taken through the steps of exploration, selection, and specification. Table 3-2 describes the criteria used in evaluating an interview between the therapist and client. In general, asking the patient's permission to move down these various levels of participation not only offers the client the opportunity to accept or reject the offer, it also makes the therapist more conscious of how planning control is shifting between the patient and the therapist. It is this consciousness that is sought in the training of therapists. Statements made to the patient offer confirmation that the therapist is aware of the changes being made.

The therapist could preface the entire interaction by stating the overall objective of having the patient contribute to the planning process and seeking his or her agreement to do so to the maximal degree possible. A sample statement could be:

> I would like you to help me so that I can help you better. I will ask you
> some questions so that we can make a plan that best meets your needs that
> we can accomplish together. I will start by asking you about the problems
> you are having in your life before asking you about what we might try to
> accomplish that will make it possible for you to see some progress. If it is
> OK with you, I will start out by asking you to tell me your own ideas in
> answer to each of the questions. If you have trouble doing that on your
> own, I will try to help you by giving you some ideas that I have learned

Table 3-2. Interview Evaluation Form: Patient Participation in Planning for Therapy

	Not Attempted	Attempted		Comments
		Incomplete	Complete	
1. Did Interviewer				
A. Introduce patient to overall procedures?				
B. Introduce exploration of concerns?				
C. Elicit at least 3 concerns?				
D. Ask for selection of priorities (either shared weights or priority?				
E. Confirm major concern(s)?				
F. Introduce exploration of goals?				
G. Introduce cooperative role in identifying goals?				
H. Elicit 3 goals?				
I. Ask for selection of one goal to pursue?				
J. Specify goal: what?				
K. setting?				
L. degree?				
2. Did interview start with open-ended question?				
3. Did interviewer ask patient's consent before moving to multiple choice, forced choice, or prescription?				
4. Did student move down steps in correct order?				
5. Did student return to open-ended questions at an appropriate time?				

from other people who have similar problems. In the long run, I can help
you best by your telling me rather than me telling you.

To the extent possible, the therapist encourages the greatest possible patient participation by asking open-ended questions, enabling the
person to function at the level of "free choice." In the step of exploration, this will mean that the patient offers several answers on his or
her own. The patient then makes the selection from those several
choices being offered. Similarly, the patient is able to freely describe the
other answers needed to specify that which has been selected in answer
to the questions asked as to "Where?" or "When?" and some measure of
degree such as "How much?" or "How well?".

To meet the other aims of generating several answers in the exploration step or in making a specific statement, the therapist may need to
provide options. One could offer several suggestions, enabling the
patient to function at the level of "multiple choice." The effect of offering several suggestions from which to choose requires the patient to
verbalize an answer in the selection step. The use of this level of participation should be prefaced by seeking agreement from the patient for
this level of participation: "Is it OK with you if I offer you some suggestions?". The term **suggestions** is defined by the fact that three
choices are offered in this exploration step. The selection step can be
carried out as before. The specification step can then be dealt with once
again by asking open questions as with "free choice." If one were to
maintain the use of "multiple choice" in the specification step, one may
again offer several suggestions from which the patient could choose
answers to the questions of "Where?" or "When?" and some measure of
degree such as "How well?" or "How much?".

Frequently several suggestions may be needed at the start. Once
given some ideas, it is easier for the patient to state freely some
answers. An example is an interview conducted with a man with recent
injury to the spinal cord in the thoracic region. He had been depressed
and had great difficulty in learning how to transfer his body from the
bed to a wheelchair although he had good strength in his arms. His
concerns and goals were not clear. When first asked about his problems
due to his injury, he made no reply. He was then offered several suggestions based on what other men with a similar injury had mentioned
when asked that same question:

THERAPIST: It is not always easy to talk about what bothers you. Is
             it OK with you if I offer you some ideas that other men
             have mentioned to me about the problems they had
             after having an injury to the spinal cord?
PATIENT: OK

THERAPIST: Other men have mentioned that they are concerned about their getting around, being able to control their urine and stay healthy, and 'not being the man they were before'.

PATIENT: Yes, I'm not the man I was before. What really bothers me is that I used to be a strong man. I was the strongest looking person at my health club. When I was a kid, I used to be beaten up by the other kids on my neighborhood. Now that I am in a wheelchair, I'm afraid that people will think that I'm weak and attack me.

This interaction started with "free choice" as to concerns but then moved to "multiple choice." When offered several suggestions, he selected one but actually generated his own answer. One of the suggestions was broad enough to provide him with a cue for his rather unexpected individualistic concern. There was now a much better basis for developing a goal statement that was meaningful to him.

Another example is that of a man with expressive aphasia who could express his ideas only by pointing. He was offered a recommendation by his therapist to follow the progress he had made in dressing himself. She asked his agreement to do more about dressing his upper body, which had been his priority during the previous week. Although unable to speak, he vehemently indicated his disagreement by shaking his head. He then gestured to his upper thigh several times to indicate his interest in doing more about pulling up and down his trousers. He was apparently particularly concerned about his ability to carry out his toileting independently when he went home.

It is usually necessary to use no lower than the level of "multiple choice" in dealing with the several steps of exploration, selection, and specification of concerns or problems and goals or the other questions. An obvious exceptions is the person with cognitive difficulties and communication problems who may require a lower level of participation. It is nevertheless possible for persons with even marked difficulties in communication to participate as long as they have consistent understanding and the ability to signify "yes" or "no."

As necessary, one can then move to the next level of making a single recommendation so that the patient is acting at the level of "forced choice." It is important to note the distinction between offering several suggestions and a single recommendation. It is desirable to ask the agreement of the patient to this change by prefacing the step with the question: "Is it OK with you if I offer you a recommendation to which you could agree or disagree?" In this level of involvement, the options are not explored but a selection already made in each instance as to what the answer might be. This same level of participation can be used in relation to the specification step wherein the answers are provided to which the client can agree (or disagree) to the questions as to "Where?" or "When?" and some measure of degree such as "How well?" or "How far?". The patient is operating on the level of agreement to that which had been decided by the professional. The patient can indicate agreement or disagreement by nodding or saying "yes" or "no." In many clinical settings, this is the level of participation used. This level of participation may be considered as minimal. The aim is to move up the scale to the extent possible during the course of ongoing interaction with the patient.

An intermediate level that can be used is that of "confirmed choice." Once agreement has been achieved in answer to the recommendations made by the professional, the clinician can then ask the patient to state that which has been agreed on. The therapist can use a statement such as "I would like to make sure we are both on the same wavelength by your telling me what we have just agreed on." In a similar fashion, one should preface one's change in level of participation by asking: "Is it OK with you if you could use your own words to describe what you have agreed to?" This level of participation marks a major transition point. It is not intended that the ideas agreed on should merely be parroted but rather in some way become part of the person. A major change occurs when the person must actively produce a statement albeit not generated initially by him. It enables the patient to modify in some way the wording of the statement offered by the professional and in this way begin to own it and become more aware of its content. It is common for the statement so generated to be somewhat different from that originally recommended yet be appropriate. It is important that the new modified wording be used henceforth.

An example of the value of involving the patient in the wording of the answer to any one of the questions is particularly illustrated in answering the question regarding "What works?". The answer(s) to that question can eventually become self-instructional. One man with major difficulty in transferring from bed to wheelchair was unable to do so safely when the therapist used various instructions. When asked to contribute to the wording, he used the word "swivel" to describe the action necessary. When used henceforth, it worked!

Another example of the value of making this transition beyond mere agreement is that of an elderly man with balance problems secondary to recurrent strokes affecting his brain stem and cerebellum. He had trouble using the walker that enabled him to maintain his balance. He lived alone and this problem he agreed would limit his ability to go home. He agreed to the recommendation of his therapist that the goal would be for him to be safe in getting around. The therapist was concerned about his ability to remember to keep his feet wide enough apart to be safe in using the walker. She had tried several different means of defining the distance by showing him and actually moving his feet apart to the proper distance. He still had difficulty recalling the proper distance consistently. The therapist thought that his cognitive impairments due to multiple strokes and advanced age would preclude his learning this crucial skill. He agreed with the instruction of keeping his feet apart. It was, however, the specification of this instruction that continued to elude him.

The decision was made to try to involve him as a way of helping him to incorporate the instruction into his actions more consistently. When he was now asked to participate in specifying how far apart his feet should be, his answer was to point to the knobs at the top of the walker to help him to estimate the proper distance. He was reinforced for the idea he had just contributed and encouraged to verbalize it as he put it into effect. His balance did indeed improve. He then continued to use this idea with good effect more consistently on his own with only occasional encouragement from his therapist.

He did not contribute the strategy in its entirety. It had been recommended to him by the therapist; however, he made it work. He had modified it by participating in its specification and, thus, made the instruction more effective. It had not only been made more specific, but it had also been made more his and more likely to be recalled and followed. He helped to make the instruction fit. By virtue of the interaction and the dialogue generated about the issue, the need for a wide base had become more salient. By eliciting his participation there was this slight increment in the ability to use the strategy that was apparently sufficient in making it effective.

It should not be necessary when dealing with concerns or goals to prescribe for the patient and thus offer "no choice." When the therapist prescribes in answer to the question of concerns or goals, the likelihood of commitment of energy to the treatment program is lessened significantly. The use of prescription infers that orders are being given. An order seeks to control the action of the other person without any opportunity to consider the actions. It might be appropriate to use this level in case of an emergency. It is usually not necessary to act on this level in dealing with the sort of problem being described in this book. The use of terms such as compliance or noncompliance betrays a lack of awareness of what could be a more optimal interaction in dealing with rehabilitation issues. Yet it is common, even with patients well able to speak for themselves, to be told by the professional not only the nature of their problem but to be given goals and assigned treatments without the opportunity for explicit agreement or any higher level of contribution. It is the premise of this book that it is far more useful to seek a greater degree of participation that can then lead to more likely adherence to the plans so generated. If it becomes necessary to use prescription, the therapist may preface this last step in the level of participation by seeking agreement: "Is it OK with you if I tell you what to do?"

It is surprising to many professionals, particularly when relatively new to the field, how well patients do in generating their own answers to the planning questions when given the opportunity to do so. It is sometimes difficult for therapists to give the patient enough time to do this. Each therapist must develop a level of tolerance for personal anxiety before intervening by moving down the scale and offering suggestions or recommendations and thus taking a greater role for planning than may actually be necessary. As one moves down the scale, more answers arise from the therapist and less commitment comes from the patient toward achieving the program plans. The more the patients are made knowledgeable about the answers by hearing them for themselves, the more the effect on them.

In evaluating the level of participation, the therapist can set objectives for the answers for each of the planning questions. For example, one may choose to involve the patient at the start of any ongoing interaction by encouraging a particular level of participation in reference to the question regarding concerns and another level in reference to the question of goals. One may seek to have the patient speak to the question about concerns at least at a "multiple choice" level and in reference to the question as to goals at least at a "forced choice" level. Only later in the review stage, one may choose to introduce patient participation in reference to the questions as to "outcomes" and at the "forced choice" level. It may take somewhat more experience encompassing several cycles before the patient is able to address the question "What worked?" at better than a "forced choice" level. One can thus specify objectives in reference to patient participation in the planning/treatment process just as one can specify objectives in reference to the clinical goals in areas such as mobility or communication. It is the premise of this book that achievement of the clinical goals will be enhanced by the attention paid to optimizing patient participation and ownership in the entire set of questions.

INTEGRATION INTO THE CLINICAL SETTING

We have reviewed the planning questions and a scale describing the level of participation achieved in answering them. The planning process schedule in most in-patient rehabilitation programs includes normal weekly or bi-weekly team meetings that serve as a checkpoint. This provides the occasion for review of the outcomes and what may have worked before revising the plan. A format for involving the patient in the team meeting is discussed in Chapter 4. The remainder of this chapter describes the application of the planning process directly within the clinical therapy session.

An example of the way the entire set of questions can be integrated into the clinical process is illustrated by a therapy session with a woman with a large defect in her skull following removal of hemorrhage in her right frontal lobe. She was trying to learn how to push her wheelchair to maintain her movement forward despite marked left field defect and neglect. The therapist was instructing her to push with her right foot and then push with the hand on the wheelchair rim. It was not working well. Instead of persisting, it was possible to develop a plan that was then implemented immediately with substantial success demonstrable during the session itself.

THERAPIST: We are tying to help you to get your wheelchair to move. Would you agree that is something you want to do?

PATIENT: I would rather get out of it. [voice low]

THERAPIST: I appreciate that you would rather get out of the chair. Would you agree for now that it would be helpful for you to get around even though you are using the chair?

PATIENT: OK. I'll try. [voice low and answer delayed]

THERAPIST: Would you agree that we want the wheelchair to move forward on a straight line? You can watch me. I will be straight in front of you.

PATIENT: OK

THERAPIST: Would you put into your own words what we agreed to do?

PATIENT: [No answer]

THERAPIST: It could help if you would push with your foot and then push the wheel of the chair. Would you agree to push with your foot?

PATIENT: OK

THERAPIST: Would you put into your own words what you agreed to do?

PATIENT: Plant my foot. [voice low and answer delayed]
THERAPIST: That's a good way to say it 'plant your foot'. [Patient
            now begins to plant her foot but was not able to then
            push the rim of the wheel in the proper sequence.]
THERAPIST: You seem to have trouble in doing one thing after the
            other. Do you agree?
PATIENT: [Nods]
THERAPIST: Can I give you the sequence?
PATIENT: [Nods]
THERAPIST: First you need to plant your foot and then push the
            wheel. Is that OK?
PATIENT: [She now carried out the sequence but only once
            before again going to the left.]
THERAPIST: You did that well. You planted your foot and then
            pushed the wheel. I will stand in front of you so that
            you can see when you are going straight. Let's try
            again. [Patient uses the sequence correctly. She now
            begins to really plant her right foot onto the ground
            slightly ahead of her. This gives her purchase on the
            floor with some forward movement occurring when she
            pushes on the rim of the wheelchair.]
THERAPIST: You are moving faster and straighter. Do you agree? It
            seems to help when you plant the foot first and then
            push the wheel. Do you agree?
PATIENT: [Nods]

This interaction occurred during the therapy session lasting about
15 minutes. To recapitulate the activities, it started with seeking the
patient's agreement to the recommended goal. The patient then
expressed her disagreement and her feelings about the goal, but, after
having received recognition for her feeling, she was nevertheless willing to agree to working on it. The goal then was further specified with
patient agreement ("moving forward on a straight line with me in
front"). The question as to "How well?" was specified as "on a straight
line" and some measure of it being met by virtue of the person standing in front. In dealing with the goal, it was not possible to move up
the scale beyond the level of "forced choice" although an attempt was
made to move to "confirmed choice." The next portion of the plan to
be decided related to the methods to be used. Her agreement was
sought to using the recommended instructions. Although agreement
was achieved, it would clearly be desirable to move up the scale to
"confirmed choice." That was achieved when the patient now changed

the wording of the instruction. In doing so, she had solved a problem that the therapist had not even been aware of. That is, the therapist had been inadvertently using the verb push for both aspects of the instruction. Actually, the patient was correct in emphasizing the need to maintain the position of the foot by planting it. The patient's contribution seemed to help solve the problem of keeping the wheelchair in a straight line. The issue remained of the two-part instruction. That was handled by getting the patient's agreement to specifying the sequence. As the patient used the sequence, it was clear that she had begun to carry out the instruction, now a shared one, with much greater force and greater success. At the end of this short session, the therapist reviewed what had been accomplished and what had worked.

It was important in this interaction to review with the patient the appropriateness of the goal as well as the means by which the goal was to be achieved. Interesting was the fact that the goal was not one the patient would have chosen but was willing to work toward at least temporarily. Only after the goal had been agreed on was it useful to address the issue of means. Given the difficulty the patient was having, it was appropriate to once again review the goal now somewhat more specified and secure after gaining her agreement to the goal. It is not always necessary to recapitulate the entire set of questions at any one time. It is helpful to recognize that there is an appropriate pairing of the questions. One can ask about goals most usefully if coupled to concerns or problems. One can ask about outcomes most usefully when coupled to goals and about methods when coupled to outcomes.

In the case just described, the next interaction at the start of a new therapy session might usefully review the outcomes and the methods that worked during the previous session. The clinician could choose to continue to work at the level of "forced choice" seeking merely agreement to a new goal for the upcoming session. "Confirmed choice" was achieved during the previous session to good effect in reference to the instructions or methods used. The therapist might try to reach a higher level of participation in relation to the means to be used in this upcoming session. One could elect to use "multiple choice" by offering several ideas from which the patient could select, thus ensuring verbalization of the instructions, or even strive with an open-ended question to seek to have the patient recall on her own the instructions that were helpful. As with the interaction just described in detail, it may be necessary only to review the goals at the start and outcomes at the end of the session while reviewing the means more often and right at the time she accomplished even a part of the total task. The therapist thus is monitoring the plan regarding the level of participation and the planning questions to be addressed along with the plan for patient's use of the wheelchair. It was the awareness of the therapist in implementing the issue of participation that enabled progress to occur in wheelchair control.

This same patient the next day was lying in bed. Rather than recommending a goal ("forced choice") for this new session, she was offered several suggestions ("multiple choice") from which to choose. She for the first time was willing to verbalize her own goal. The previous day, before the episode described above, she had not been willing to participate on this higher level in respect to the transfer issue. She selected "getting out of bed into the wheelchair" when also offered the choice of "exercising in bed" or "getting to sit up." Because she was lying in bed, the first goal, when now given a "forced choice," was her agreement to "roll over." The method for her to use to accomplish this was generated by an open-ended question: "How would you be able to roll over?" She then was able to speak for herself and reply "use the bed rail." She then did so on her own. Throughout the session she was offered the opportunity to select from several suggestions as to how to get herself to transfer now that she was sitting on the edge of the bed. She selected "scoot" from the other suggestions, which included "stand up and pivot" as well. When she was not able to scoot the entire distance necessary, she was able to instruct the therapist to "help me scoot." By instructing the therapist aloud, she was also instructing herself. By operating under the patient's direction, the desired shift had occurred. Although the action could not be carried out in its entirety by the patient alone, the help provided by the other person was under her direction. Ultimately the instruction being given to the other was also being given by the patient to herself.

This episode illustrates the progress made in generalizing the level of participation achieved during the previous episode dealing with wheelchair mobility. The patient had become better able to participate in goal setting and defining the means to be used in this area of her transfer from bed to chair in a way that she had not done the previous day when trying to deal with this same issue. The experience she had in dealing with her wheelchair control had apparently contributed to her sense of self and strengthened her commitment to dealing with other matters as well.

In general, when a person is asked about what worked immediately after the action had been taken, after describing the action and thus becoming more aware, the person can put it into effect repeatedly during the session itself. This was useful with a man who had difficulty learning to put his affected arm into his sleeve first in putting on his shirt. Time spent in reviewing the procedures just used in the context of their use was crucial according to one therapist. She found it became less necessary for her to reinforce the actions. She found that the patient began quite soon to give himself the instructions at first by verbalizing them as he carried them out and then carrying out the actions independently having apparently internalized the instructions. She found that the experience of becoming more aware of his own actions also helped the man set his own goals and recognize his own accomplishments. Willingness to address one's problems in a frank fashion also began to occur. The therapist found that the entire process of planning could go on within the session with the patient contributing ideas freely. The time invested earlier in the course of the recurrent therapy sessions now began to pay dividends not only in terms of results but also in terms of efficiency.

Involving patients as active participants can also make more efficient the transfer of information when there might be need for dealing with a number of different therapists. Patients learning how to manage themselves after knee surgery agreed to recommended goal of "ambulating with an assistive device" when discharged home. To accomplish this long-term goal, it was necessary to set short-term goals regarding the range of motion at the knee each day. This could be easily measured with the results clearly understood by the patient. The daily status could be recorded on a sheet of paper by the patient at the end of each day. By so doing, the patient was functioning at the level of "confirmed agreement" when she wrote that which had been dictated by the therapist. Further participation in actually reading the result from the instrument used to measure range of motion and then writing it down would have the patient operating at an even higher level of participation analogous to making a "free choice" in answer to the open-ended question as to "What is the range of motion?". The record brought by the patient to the next day's group session was a basis for communication when it was necessary for the patient to work with different therapists. The patient became the carrier of the information. In so doing, not only was there the opportunity to ensure that the various therapists were kept abreast of the status, but the patient could now reinforce herself about her progress. Every attempt possible was made to have the patient "in the loop."

An occupational therapist recalls vividly the break-through experience of enabling a teenager with recent cord injury and paraplegia to learn about himself in the context of a therapy session. He was depressed and unwilling to participate in learning how to control his trunk although he had the muscles available to do so. However, he was able to make progress when asked about the games he liked to play. He mentioned badminton and then while trying to swing the racket he indeed began to control his trunk. When asked about the progress he had made, he was at first unable to describe it. The therapist recommended the idea that he was "no longer walking up with his hands to straighten himself up." He could agree to this description. Once he was able to measure for himself the results that had occurred, he was then better able to address subsequent questions about goals for the next session incorporating the control of the trunk muscles in leaning over to carry out his dressing.

Eliciting answers to the question as to what actions may have helped is particularly valuable as an integral part of the clinical sessions. The description of the actions taken should be kept simple because they must ultimately be translatable into self-instructions. They need to be described in terms that the patient can use to instruct himself. For example, a man with hemiplegia stood successfully within the parallel bars for the first time. When he could not respond on a "free choice" level in answer to an open-ended question, he was offered several suggestions that were deliberately couched in terms of relatively specific instructions. He chose "locking my knee" and also another that had been suggested, namely, "holding on with my arms." He then rather surprisingly mentioned freely on his own "knowing what I was trying to do." All these actions could be used again in the effort to improve his walking. In addition, the last statement, one that he had made on his own, dealt with the more general principle of being clear about his goals. This was an action the patient could apply to a far larger set of problems than merely one of walking, although the idea arose in the context of the specific situation of learning to walk. In this way, an awareness arises not only of some of the answers to the questions but also an awareness of the value of asking the question itself.

The process of increased ownership of strategies was also illustrated in another case. A woman with long-standing right-sided weakness caused by a stroke had been unable to transfer out of bed without the aid of her husband. Her goal she stated on her own to be to "get in and out of bed from my wheelchair without any help from my husband." On her own, she had stated a goal that met the criteria of specificity. In doing this multistep procedure she was able to perform the steps in the correct order. She would use the instruction: "First, slide forward, second straighten out my leg, third get up." She was able to carry out the first step in sliding forward in her chair to bring her weight more directly over her legs. However, she continued to have difficulty in pulling herself to a standing position. She could not straighten her leg out sufficiently to pull herself up. In addition to her limb weakness, old surgery to her unaffected knee prevented full range of motion. It was clearly necessary for her to somehow compensate for this problem by increasing the ability to pull herself up using the arm strength that remained in the unaffected arm. The instruction given her to use was to "lift up." It had not been sufficient to bring about the result she had committed herself to achieving. It was necessary to use every ounce of her energy to this effort.

She was given the recommendation of instructing her husband "lift" when she was ready to rise up. He would then raise her to a standing position but only after repeating her instruction. They agreed to this recommendation. However, when first putting it into practice, she used her own word by saying "up" rather than "lift" as had been recommended. Although she had given the instruction, it had not been done with any force behind it. She had nevertheless made the important step that she was no longer being lifted without her participation. The husband awaiting her instruction was important because he acted on it when feeding it back to her; she was indeed giving herself the instruction along with giving it to her husband. At first, she was primarily giving the instruction to her husband rather than commanding herself. After a number of trials, she was giving the instruction to herself with commitment of the energy required to overcome the difficulty with her knee. She would order "UP!" The additional increment by virtue of her phrasing of the command and her commitment of energy to its use was actually bringing her to a standing position. She had met her goal and was pleased with herself. When asked further about what she did to bring about the result, she stated "I was afraid I would fall. I could see that I could do it and I was the one who really could get it to happen." Rather than continuing to order herself with the explosive loud command "UP!" she now performed the action without the need to say it aloud. She now was prepared to set a new goal to increase her ability to walk. She stated on her own her method of doing so would be to instruct herself by the order with which she would go about it with "cane first, then left (affected) leg and then right (unaffected) leg."

This case illustrates the transfer of the level of participation entirely to the patient rather than the other person. She had taken full control of her herself and was now commanding herself to ensure the greatest possible commitment of energy. It is the opposite of the situation wherein she was commanded by another. It also illustrates the generalization possible in using the strategy helpful in dealing with a multistep procedure, such as transfer, to perhaps an even more complex sequence such as walking.

PLANNING FOR ONESELF III

What Are the Outcomes?

You should start by applying the question to personal issues for yourself relative to the goals of this book; that is, the student/clinician acts first to do for oneself what one will later do with the patient. You should first evaluate the outcome of the educational program thus far, before redefining the problems and goals for the continuation of the educational program, including a time line for oneself for re-evaluation. The student may, like the patient, have set goals that are somewhat different from those set out by the faculty of any course one is taking. It is those personal goals that are being evaluated and revised.

In addressing the question of what results you have achieved in relation to your previous goals, you should follow the pattern already established. Explore several outcomes before selecting the outcome about which you feel the best or the one that you remember the best and specify that particular outcome. The actual results specified should meet the criteria for specificity; that is, the statement as to outcome would include *what* was achieved, *where* or *when* it happened, and *to what degree*. As a result of defining outcomes, remaining concerns and appropriate goals for the future will become clearer. The rate of accomplishment may have been greater than expected or less, and so the time line may change. Once concerns have been identified, existing goals may need to be modified in some way or a new goal may need to be created.

One student who successively carried out this cyclical process illustrated the relationship between the original concerns and the goals, the relationship of outcomes to goals, and the establishment of new goals in relation to new concerns. Her major concern during the early portion of her first clinical rotation was "being able to ask appropriate questions during the clinical interview to the extent of getting a specific goal." To deal with this concern, she set a goal of "getting a specific goal during three remaining interviews without feeling awkward and without someone having to give me direction."

When reviewing the outcomes, she described herself as "successful in controlling the direction of the conversation during the last interview to the extent of getting a specific goal." She succeeded at reaching the goal about which she had been concerned. Now that she was more secure about the technical aspects, she had a new concern—when to start this process: "I don't feel sure about when to initiate this goal-planning process with a patient." Her aim during her next clinical rotation was to experiment with the timing to become clearer about how to use this process most effectively.

When reviewing her second clinical rotation, this same student described herself as "better able to ask appropriate questions and more comfortable during the interview." Her concern now dealt with integrating the approach so that it was flexible and compatible with herself. Many students move in this way from more technical concerns to the more abstract concerns.

Review the goals you listed for yourself in the exercise at the end of Chapter 2. Now use the format described in Table 3-3 (PPS-2) to evaluate your results in dealing with those personal professional concerns and goals relative to mastering the approach described in this book. Then list the concerns that remain or have newly arisen. List your goals for the next block of time and specify at least one of them. You can use this same format to re-evaluate your performance in an ongoing way throughout your professional career. Remember that you don't have to

---

Table 3-3. Program Planning Sheet 2 (PPS-2)

Name _____   Date _____

Therapist _____

1. **What results have you achieved?** (List at least 3.) Select your best result with asterisk and have that statement meet the 4 criteria of "specificity."

2. **What problems do you have? What questions do you have?** (List at least 3.) Select your greatest concern with an asterisk and have that statement meet the 3 criteria of "specificity."

3. **What would you like to see accomplished that would make you feel that you are making some progress in dealing with your greatest concern?** (List 3 and specify the most important one with 3 criteria.)

use the participation line when working on your own personal goals. Be sure the exercise is expressed in personal terms, using personal pronouns. Try to do the exercise on your own first; then if you need some help or suggestions from others, you may turn to examples of what other students have done as illustrated in Tables 3-4 and 3-5.

Table 3-4. Student Use of Form 2, Completed after a Patient Interview, during a Part-Time Clinical Rotation

1. **What results have you achieved?** (List at least 3.) Select your best result with an asterisk and have that statement meet the criteria of "specificity."
   1. I have learned when open-ended questions, suggestions, recommendations, and prescriptions are appropriate during an interview.
   2. I have learned how to differentiate between a goal and a means during an interview.
   *3. I have learned how to interview a patient following the guidelines learned in my clinical problem-solving class, in clinic, during regular therapy time, to the degree that when I interview patients in the clinic they can generate 3 concerns, a main concern, 3 goals, and a specific goal which is relevant to the main concern.

2. **What problems do you have now? What questions do you have?** (List at least 3.) Select your greatest concern with an asterisk and have that statement meet the criteria of "specificity."
   1. I am concerned that I do not yet have enough medical knowledge to always know whether the goals set by a patient are within reason.
   *2. I would like to learn how to respond to a patient during an interview when he sets a goal that is in all likelihood not attainable, to the degree that I can get him to set a short-term goal that is reasonable.
   3. I would like to learn what to do if, during an interview, none of the goals the patient is concerned with are things that relate to therapy.

3. **What would you like to see accomplished which would make you feel that you are making some progress in dealing with your gretest concern?** (List 3 and specify 1.)
   1. That I am realistic in response to an unobtainable goal.
   2. That I not reject a patient's goal if it appears to be unobtainable.
   *3. That if a patient states an unobtainable goal, I can redirect him toward making a goal that is obtainable, but still let him make the goal in the clinic where he is receiving therapy to the degree that his goal is within reason based on his medical situation.

Time line: By the end of this semester

Table 3-5. Illustration of the Use of Form 2 by a Student after Several Patient Interviews

---

1. **What results have you achieved?** (List at least 3.) Select your best result with an asterisk and have that statement meet the criteria of specificity.
   1. I have developed the ability to elicit important concerns from patients.
   2. I have developed the ability to convert concerns into goals that meet the criteria of specificity.
   *3. I have developed the ability to prioritize goals using the weight-sharing system with patients in occupational therapy practice when I interview them during therapy.

2. **What problems do you have? What questions do you have?** (List at least 3.) Select your greatest concern with an asterisk and have that statement meet the criteria of specificity.
   *1. I have difficulty explaining the weight-sharing system to patients so that they understand the process in a short period of time (less than 2 minutes) in a clinical setting.
   2. What are the results of writing goals this way versus other methods (i.e., are patients more motivated for treatment)?
   3. How do I use this method to elicit appropriate goals from patients who are unrealistic in their expectations?

3. **What would you like to see accomplished that would make you feel that you are making some progress in dealing with your greatest concern?** (List 3 and specify 1.)
   *1. I would like to be able to develop 3 specific methods of explaining the weight-sharing system that can be used with patients on my next affiliation.
   2. I would like to be able to redirect patients to develop realistic goals.
   3. I would like to be able to elicit goals from patients and form them to meet the criteria of specificity in a short amount of time.

Time line: By the end of my spring affiliation

Note that the outstanding achievement in the student's mind has an asterisk, and it is specified to four criteria (what, where, when, degree). The concern and goal selected as primary are specified to three criteria (what, where, when, degree) as discussed in Chapter 2. Time lines are also specified. The goal in Table 3-4 is somewhat vague in terms of degree, but it is still acceptable. Note the goal statement at the end of Table 3-4 meets the three criteria of specificity but not in the usual order.

What Works?

The application of the process for oneself thus far has been to use the basic question of concerns at the end of Chapter 1 and to review concerns and set goals at the end of Chapter 2. Once you have set goals, you can perform the review process to measure outcome in relation to the initial set of goals, reconsider concerns, and revise the goals. Three of the basic questions have been addressed, some more than once.

The basic Program Planning Sheet (PPS) has become progressively more complex to reflect the use of the successive planning questions. Once again, you can now add to the planning process the use of the question as to means. PPS-3 in Table 3-6 completes the formats that can be used to document the process of ongoing planning. For the first time, the question "What worked?" has been incorporated into the planning process.

Table 3-6. Program Planning Sheet 3 (PPS-3)

Name _____   Date _____

                                                 Therapist _____

1. **What results have you achieved?** (List at least 3.) Select your best result with asterisk and have that statement meet the criteria of "specificity."

   Level of participation _____
2. **What actions did you take that may have helped to bring about those results?** (List at least 3.) Select what you feel was most helpful and meet the criteria of "specificity" for that statement using an asterisk.

   Level of participation _____
3. **What problems do you have now? What questions do you have?** (List at least 3.) Select your greatest concern with an asterisk and have that statement meet the criteria of "specificity."

   Level of participation _____

(Continued)

Table 3-6. (Continued)

4. **What would you like to see accomplished that would make you feel that you are making some progress in dealing with your greatest concern?** (List 3.)

5. **What is your plan?**
   A. **GOAL** (Please be specific)
      What?
      Setting?
      To what degree?
   B. **MEANS** (identify from those actions which may have worked in 2 above)
   C. **Time line**

Level of participation _____

In exploring the question of means, it is again important to list at least three aspects before selecting one that seems the most important, as making the greatest contribution. Then specify it meeting whatever criterion you wish to use. It is generally useful to make it as specific as possible so that you can be clear about how you accomplished something. You can specify it to meet the 4-point criterion; that is, to describe not only *what* but *where* and *when* and *to what degree.* The other aspect to keep in mind about the use of the answers to this question is that those arising in the context of the outcomes already achieved can now also be used as part of the plan for the future. The plan in the fifth section of the PPS-3 contains all three components: the goal, the means, and the time line.

With the use of the format found in Table 3-6, several therapists in training evaluated their performance in carrying out several interviews with patients. The selected outcome for one student was "learning during the interview that my patient was more insightful than I thought." In reference to that outcome, the student/therapist explored this new question as to what may have helped to bring about the result.

The following answers arose out of the use of the question as to "What worked?": "giving the patient control," "using the format of the structured interview process," and "focusing on patient activities rather than pain." When the therapist was asked to select the activity that she contributed the most, she chose "using the format of the structured interview process." She stated: "I knew what I was doing." The emphasis in this exercise was to enhance the therapist's sense of control by helping her focus on what she did that may have brought about the result. Later, when the question as to what works is applied to patients, the emphasis will be on what the patient did that contributed to bring about the results achieved.

A therapist in an in-service training program described her achievements in the application of this approach to patient care as follows: "Patients will generally set their own goals. I can get more of a measurable achievement. I'm more aware of doing things in a logical, quantitative way." The outcome most meaningful was "I wasn't stuck as much in a rut. I'm trying new things." In answer to the question as to what worked, she reported, "I discussed the new methods with my classmates. I kept an open mind. I watched the instructor work with patients." When asked what did *you* do to help bring about the results? She answered, "I practiced on my own." Here again, the answers to the questions are in relation to *your* actions. Personalizing the answers concerning your own actions can help you enable patients to do the same.

Tables 3-7, 3-8, and 3-9 illustrate the application of all five questions now using the expanded PPS-3. Note the relationships among the various parts of these samples. Each new section flows from the answers to the previous question. Note also the way the means generated earlier in the context of the outcome (Question 2) can now be written as the means part of the plan (Question 5).

Table 3-7. Example of Student Use, at the End of a Week of Full-Time Clinical Study, of PPS-3 Concerning Her Own Interests

1. What results have you achieved?
   - A. I have been more successful in terms of controlling the direction of conversation during the patient interview for the duration of the interview.
   - B. I feel that I am now able to document and understand patient's concerns/goals while conducting the interview so that I can gather appropriate information related to the patient's problem.
   - *C. I was able to work with the patient (we were a team) during an interview at the hospital in the time allotted (20 minutes).

2. What actions/means were used to produce those results?
   - A. I had several opportunities to observe a therapist demonstrate relevant skills while working with patients.
   - *B. It was helpful that I was responsible for developing SOAP notes (goal statements) in the clinic during my rotation for at least one patient each day on my own.

Table 3-7. (Continued)

C. It was helpful to interact with patient and therapists daily for a week.

3. What problems do you still have?
   * A. I still have some trouble thinking of appropriate questions to ask during the interview so that I feel comfortable during the interview.
   B. I don't know enough about therapy at this point.
   C. I feel inexperienced talking to patients.

4. What are your goals?
   A. Talk more with patients
   B. Study therapy methods
   * C. Conduct an interview using questions
   During my next clinical experience
   To the degree that both patient and I feel that we have set meaningful goals for therapy

5. What is your plan?
   Goal: Conduct several interviews with a patient in clinic and generate a goal acceptable to both patient and me without feeling uncomfortable during the interview
   Means: Practice by being responsible for writing SOAP notes.
   Watch others interview patients.
   Get feedback from others when I interview.
   Time line: By the end of my next full-time clinical experience

Table 3-8. Example of Student Use of Form PPS-3

1. What results have you achieved?
   * A. Able to ask more appropriate, direct questions during interview in clinic so that PPS-3 was completed in 20 minutes
   B. Able to manage time allotted
   C. Able to encourage patient without leading him

2. What actions helped to bring about those results?
   * A. I practiced the process with family and friends as often as possible after class to the degree that I had the form memorized
   B. Read patient's history before interview
   C. Reviewed previous interviews and studied my mistakes

3. What problems remain?
   A. Still feel uncomfortable interviewing patients
   B. Have problems isolating a specific goal
   * C. Dealing with a variety of patient concerns in clinical settings so that I feel comfortable

4. What would you like to see yourself accomplishing in the future which would make you feel that you were making progress in dealing with your concerns?

Table 3-8. (Continued)

A. I would like to be able to complete an initial interview in 15 minutes or less.

*B. I would like to interview several patients with different problems in clinic and feel comfortable no matter what the problem.

C. I would like to be able to isolate one specific goal and specify it.

5. What is your plan?

Goal: Interview any patient in a hospital or clinical setting and generate a specific goal in 15 minutes or less with maximum patient participation.

Means: Practice interviewing as often as possible with anyone who is willing wherever possible and completing each interview within 20 minutes.

By when: By the end of summer affiliation

Table 3-9. Example of Student Assessment of His Own Educational Plans Relative to Program Planning with Patients

---

1. What results have you achieved?

*A. I understand the importance of using open-ended questions during the interview, in a clinical setting, to the extent that I can achieve more patient participation.

B. I gained more practical experience in the interview process to the extent that I feel more comfortable.

C. I have gained more confidence in my ability to conduct an interview with a patient in clinic so that I feel comfortable.

2. What actions helped bring about these results?

A. Listening to interviews done by other therapists

*B. Practicing interviewing with several patients, in clinic, during earlier clinical affiliations, as often as possible

C. Practicing with students, friends, and family, in class, at home, on weekends, as often as possible

3. What problems remain?

A. I still feel inexperienced.

*B. Can I really help patients establish functional goals, during an interview, in clinic, to the degree that they are realistic and specific?

C. Can I deal effectively with uncooperative patients?

4. What would you like to see happen?

A. Do interviews that result in meaningful goal writing

B. Successfully interview other health professionals

*C. Perform several interviews with patients in a clinical setting so that the total plan is written to the satisfaction of both the patient and myself

---

Table 3-9. (Continued)

---

5. What is your plan?

Goal: Complete several patient *plans* in clinic so that both of us are satisfied

Means: Practice, practice, practice with different patients every day during the therapy sessions

By when: The end of the summer clinicals

....

A word needs to be said about flexibility. A student/therapist reported on the success she had integrating the various questions of the planning process into her daily contact with her patients during her summer rotations. She found her patients accepting readily her questions about their problems. She would ask in a "straightforward way and her clients would tell her about their problems. She could then focus them and help them be specific about goals.

She would use the questions in a conversational way. For example, while she was ranging the patient's limbs, she would ask what the patient felt was being accomplished. She found that the patients became more enthusiastic and carried that enthusiasm over into other aspects of their lives in the hospital. She felt that what helped to bring about their participation was that the patients knew someone was listening. Using the question "What do you want to get out of therapy?" was her way of getting across the idea of setting goals. By addressing this question, the patient comes with a purpose and more often tells the therapist what he needs to accomplish in a particular session. She found people setting more reasonable goals and taking it one step at a time. She felt what worked was "asking questions rather than giving orders, giving the patients time to talk, acting as though the patient is a real partner in therapy and being specific about the goals."

....

APPLICATION TO PATIENT CARE I

Now that you have experienced the full range of planning questions in your own work, you can begin to use each of the questions with patients. The added parameter is the awareness of the degree of participation you have achieved from the patient in answering these questions. Each incorporates an increasing range of questions along with some measure of participation. You will use these forms with patients to document the degree of patient participation achieved in answering the several components of the goal statement. The score reflects the scale in Table 3-1. Note that there is no provision for "E," which reflects the level of "no choice" represented by the use of a prescription. If no score is placed, one can assume that the absence reflects that none of the levels of participation above that of prescription was used.

One aspect to patient participation is to state clearly to the patient the goals for the interview and the steps you will take for reaching those goals. As one student put it, "You start by telling the patient that you are going to explore what might be problems before then, trying to find what would be ways one could tell that those problems are being solved." The ground rules are further described in terms of hearing from patients what their concerns are and what might be some of their goals. You may tell them that you will help if they "get stuck," but it is important for them to tell you what matters to them. Some patients may be surprised to be involved in goal setting, thinking that it is the therapist's responsibility rather than theirs. In such a case, you should convey the reasons for inviting such participation as expressed throughout this book.

Do all the things discussed thus far:

1. Explore several concerns in depth or in breadth.

2. Have the patient select one chief concern (either by weighting or by simply selecting the greatest concern).

3. Explore several goals that would be indicators of progress toward alleviating that concern.

4. Have the patient select the most important or first goal to be accomplished before specifying it.

After introducing yourself and stating the purpose of the interview, the first step is to explore concerns/problems with the patient. Some students have had difficulty in asking questions regarding problems in ways that are directly applicable to a patient. For example, a patient first described his concern as not being able to walk. When he denied any other problems, the next question continuing the exploration step could have been "What might be keeping you from walking?" rather than giving up on exploring problems at that point.

There are two aspects to the interview as documented on the forms provided. One is the answers to the planning questions that can later be used for writing notes in the clinical record. The other is the process or method by which the answers are generated. The level of participation is an important part of this second aspect. It can tell you how much the answers on the form are the patient's and thus their strength or value in planning. Be aware of the level of participation as the interview progresses. Each time you feel you need to change the level of participation, notify the patient of the change and seek his or her agreement to that change before proceeding. For example, you could ask "Is it OK with you if I give you some suggestions?" as the entry to provid-

ing the patient with the several choices. This respects the patient's dignity and alerts you to what you are doing during the interview.

The final component of the basic form (PPS-1) is the recording of
the level of patient participation in the development of each aspect of
the specified goal. Simply circle A, B, C, or D to indicate the *lowest* level
of patient participation needed in the final specification of the goal. If
it is necessary to move to "multiple choice," then the goal statement is
scored at that level of participation even if only one portion of the goals
statement required that degree of therapist contribution. The level of
participation may be important in evaluating the outcome at a later
date. When using more advanced formats for planning, the ABCD scale
will be abandoned for just a line to document the actual level of participation.

Examples of therapist interviews of patients are found in Tables 3-
10 and 3-11. Table 3-11 shows the use of a weighting procedure to

---

Table 3-10. Example of Use of PPS-1 with a Patient, by a Student, Sections on Concerns and Goals

Patient _____   Date _____

                                            Therapist _____

PROGRAM PLANNING SHEET 1

1. What are your concerns?
    1. I cannot play golf once a week with my friends like I did a year ago
       because holding a golf club in my hand is so painful.
    2. I cannot spread mayonnaise on bread, open a jar or milk carton
       when I want to eat, without someone helping me.
  *3. I cannot get dressed without help from my wife.

2. What is your greatest concern?
   I can't get dressed by myself.

3. Check out: __*_*__ agreed _____ confirmed

4. What do you want to see happen? What would make you feel that you
   are making progress in relation to your major concern? What are your
   goals?
    1. I want to be able to put on my socks by myself.
    2. I want to be able to put on my pants by myself.
  *3. I want to be able to put on my shirt without help.

5. What is your specific goal?
    Ⓐ B C D   What: Put on my shirt
    Ⓐ B C D   Setting: In the morning
    A Ⓑ C D   Degree: In less than 10 minutes and without help

---

Table 3-11. Example of an Interview Done by an Occupational Therapist

Patient _____   Date _____8-5-98_____

Therapist _____

1. What are your concerns?
   1. Being able to dress myself
   2. Like to know if I can return to hair dressing if I want
   3. Can I grasp a glass? Can I grasp things with my fingers?
   4. Will I become depressed?
   5. Will the pain continue or subside?
   6. Could the arm eventually "flare up" (e.g., arthritis)?
   7. Afraid to drive at night

2. What are your major concerns?
   0   0 = 0 mental attitude
      0   3 = 3 arm flare-up
   3 3   = 6 pain
   Pain confirmed as chief concern.

3. What are your goals?
   *1. That I could go to sleep at night and sleep well without drugs
   2. That I could tolerate pain for longer periods of time (e.g., while
      I grip a broom and sweep the kitchen floor or while ironing)*
   3. That I could tolerate massage of my fingers (e.g., tolerate force of
      shower water on my hand)*

4. What is your first goal?
   (A) B C D   What: A good night's rest
   (A) B C D   Setting: At home
   A (B) C D   Degree: Straight through without disturbance from
                               my fingers

....

* Examples were elicited when I asked her for functional examples.

select from a larger number of concerns than usually elicited. It concerns a 41-year-old female hairdresser who sustained a near amputation of the left upper extremity above the elbow with fracture at the junction of the distal and middle third of the humerus. She was initially seen by a hand therapist at bedside for fabrication of a volar static wrist splint. She was wearing a humeral external fixator at the time of the interview. Whenever she did not understand a question, she asked the therapist to give her examples. She did not, however, use the examples for her answers and was very verbal during the interview. A two-step process was used to select the priorities. Because there were a large number to start, the therapist asked her to select three priorities and then used a weighting procedure to identify the one priority area.

One important stimulus to the process of encouraging patient participation is providing evidence that the patient's statements are being heard. A useful technique for doing this is to record patient statements on a pad of paper in full view of the patient, repeating aloud what you are writing as you write it. This provides direct evidence that the patient is being heard. This procedure also provides a record of the interview for later analysis or discussion.

Now that you have completed a patient interview leading to a goal, the next step is to review and revise this initial plan, which will be done at the end of Chapter 4.

Part 2

Implementation

In Part One of this book, we described the planning process starting with the overall plan, then recapitulating the planning procedures in greater detail: the planning questions and the measurement of the degree to which the primary participants were enabled to participate in that process. At the end of each chapter, the third component of any planning process was exemplified in the evaluation of the process. The exercises at the end of each chapter offered an additional opportunity for practice in the implementation of the process both for you in dealing with your own educational program in using this book and in implementation with a patient.

Part Two discusses the implementation process in greater detail and variety. Chapter 4 (Coordinated Planning) describes the implementation within the usual interdisciplinary team planning structure. The application to patient care exercises have two aspects. Application to Patient Care II continues with the participation of the patient in the review/revision process to complete the cycle started in the earlier exercise at the end of Chapter 3. Application to Patient Care III marks the opportunity to design the application of the participatory planning system to a programmatic level.

Chapter 5 (Integration in the Clinical Setting) illustrates the implementation of the participatory planning process in a variety of clinical situations. Its use in the clinical record is exemplified in terms of the SOAP note and other types of documentation requirements. It shows its implementation within groups as well as other types of formats. Application to Patient Care IV completes the process of implementation at a programmatic level by carrying out the review and feedback step.

Chapter 6 (Educational Programs) describes the use of the planning process in a variety of educational formats including an ongoing process of staff development. Each of the chapters in this second part also replicates the structure of the overall planning process with identification of the problem, the procedures, and methods for evaluation.

Chapter 4

Coordinated Planning

THE GOALS OF THE CHAPTER

This chapter deals with the format for introducing the patient and family into the interdisciplinary team structure used in many rehabilitation settings. The team planning structure provides an opportunity for the coordination of what is sometimes a relatively comprehensive approach to persons with complex needs. Rather than a single professional interacting with the patient or family, the size of the team is expanded to include additional professionals. Coordination of this enlarged team is necessary. The planning questions described in the earlier chapters and a scale used for measuring patient participation in answering the planning can all be modified. The scale for measuring patient participation can vary. The modifications to meet the constraints of the team and the time allotments as well as the type of patient problem illustrate how the basic structure can be used in response to different requirements.

The aim is for the patient and caregiver to become participants in making this effort a truly coordinated one. The team must focus on priorities organized around those of the individual characteristics of the patient. Ultimately, in light of a sometimes lengthy rehabilitation program, one objective can be for the patient or family to learn how to become coordinators. Their experience in doing so from the start can enable these primary participants to expand their role as coordinators and become more independent in that role as well as in being a planner. By the end of this chapter, you should be able to design a team planning process and its evaluation.

INTERDISCIPLINARY PLANNING

The Nature of the Problem

The team conference is the basis for the ongoing planning process involving the team of professionals in many rehabilitation settings. It has been under increasing scrutiny in terms of both costs and questionable results. For example, the membership of the team dealing with the acute rehabilitation of persons with stroke can contain as many as seven persons. One such team has assigned roles to the various members as follows. The physician has the role of dealing with the medical problems along with the role of team manager for purposes of legal responsibility for the medical necessity of certain procedures. The nurse is assigned the role of designing and carrying out the training of the patient and family in preventing recurrent strokes. An occupational therapist trains the patient and family in dealing with activities of daily living such as eating, dressing, and toileting. The physical therapist is concerned with issues of mobility such as transfers between bed and chair, wheelchair mobility, and ambulating. Often a speech therapist is assigned to deal with issues such as swallowing and speech clarity and communication, and a psychologist deals with cognitive and emotional issues. A rehabilitation care coordinator connects with third-party payers or a social worker who can also be involved with family participation and follow-up after discharge. The particular make-up of any team can vary as can the roles assigned to each of the professional disciplines.

The time allotted for meeting of such a costly group must be limited. The frequency of such meetings as well as their duration is a major concern in many rehabilitation settings. Even more important has been concern about its effectiveness. The multidisciplinary nature of the team has been modified to reflect a greater degree of coordination with the use of the term **interdisciplinary** to describe its mode of operation, impling that the team operates in a more coordinated fashion than merely a collection of professionals. In some settings, cross-training of staff has occurred to function in a transdisciplinary team enabling fewer persons to be needed.

An opportunity to make rehabilitation more cost-effective lies in modifying the planning structure to make it more effective without increasing costs. A method to do so is to enhance the coordination of these various staff. The method described here makes the planning more effective by involving the patient and family as more active participants. Their participation can create greater focus on meaningful priorities and increase the likelihood of their contributing energy to the implementation of the plans made. This new focus changes the objectives of the team meeting to incorporate not only the coordination between the various professionals but also toward bringing the patient onto the team at the time when decisions are actually being made. Time and staff are used more effectively because no increase in time is needed, but the way time is spent is improved. Every member of the planning team, regardless of other roles, would participate in this overall effort. The responsibility for ensuring such participation as assigned "patient advocate" or "coach" could be any team member. The same or some other team member can be also responsible for documenting the participation that occurred. In some settings, this task is rotated as a means of increasing the awareness of all the team members of the participation issue. At other times, one or another team member serves that role depending on interest and availability.

The need to bring the patient and family onto the team makes it necessary to have the planning activities of the team even more highly specified than when only one professional interacts with the patient. The extent to which specification occurs with resultant overall awareness of the objectives can contribute to making the entire planning process more effective. The documentation of the degree the objectives were being met also must meet the constraints of costs. Meeting this issue led to evaluation being done intrinsic to the treatment setting.

The Planning Process

The basic cyclical planning structure remains. At least two planning sessions are held during the course of an in-patient stay with at least one additional session after discharge. Another option is continuing planning meetings with the frequency depending on the intensity of services being provided. For example, one pattern has been to hold weekly meetings during the usually more intensive in-patient stay with biweekly and then monthly planning meetings to reflect a lesser intensity of ongoing services while the patient is receiving out-patient services. Governmental and other third-party payers generally require bi-weekly planning review.

The hospital-based interdisciplinary team conference described here is only an example. The frequency of planning meetings and the components of the team will vary in other settings. One such setting is long-term care where costs may be highly constrained. Yet planning and review must continue. The example should be adapted to the time constraints. Regardless of the setting, the principle remains that an opportunity to make such planning more effective lies in enlisting the energy and ideas of those most directly involved, namely, the patient and family.

Table 4-1 describes this overall structure. In the example used of an in-patient hospital-based stroke program, the length of stay has been about 21 days. This has permitted three planning sessions during that time. The first occurs within 72 hours of admission, the second 1 week later, and the third meeting just before discharge. An initial follow-up meeting is held within 2 weeks after discharge with subsequent meetings depending on the intensity of services to be provided. A different planning frequency can be designed for shorter or longer lengths of stay. For example, a program for postoperative knee and hip replacement has had a 1 week length of stay with the initial meeting on the first day and a second on the day before discharge and another 1 week after discharge. For a longer length of stay for persons with head injury,

Table 4-1. Stroke Recovery Program: Rehabilitation Patient Self-Management

	Day 1–3 Assessment	Day 4 Initial inpatient team meeting	Day 11 Interim team meeting	Day 18 Discharge team meeting	Varies Initial ambulatory team meeting	Varies Interim ambulatory meeting(s)	Varies Discharge team meeting
Activities	Rehab. plan designed	Inpatient interdisciplinary rehab. plan completed	I/P rehab. plan implemented/ reviewed/ revised	I/P rehab. plan reviewed/ revised Ambulatory rehab plan designed	Ambulatory rehab plan completed	Ambulatory rehab. plan implemented/ reviewed /revised	↑
Objectives	1. Rehab. problems identified 2. Goals established	1. Status reviewed 2. Priority goals established	1. Status established 2. New goals established	1. New status established 2. What worked established 3. New goals established	↑	↑	↑

79

a family meeting is planned within 1 week of admission to design the caregiver training plan, with another meeting in the week before discharge, and a follow-up meeting 2 weeks after discharge home.

The principle has been to maintain a recurrent planning process with the identification of short-term and long-term objectives during the initial meeting and then the opportunity to review progress and revise the initial plan at subsequent meetings. The professionals address the questions as to problems and status in their particular domain before the first of the team meetings. During that initial planning meeting, an interdisciplinary plan is formulated and short-term goals for interdisciplinary issues are determined. At the subsequent meetings, the review process asks the questions about new status or outcomes and strategies before making a new plan. The recurrent use of the appropriate planning questions contributes to the eventual goal of enabling the patient or family to become more active participants in answering the planning questions as well as becoming more aware of the questions themselves.

The planning questions are addressed as usual. However, the requirement to develop a coordinated interdisciplinary plan at the initial team meeting changes the way the questions are answered. During the initial assessment before the first of the team meetings, each of the appropriate therapists addresses the question "What is the problem?". The purpose of this question is to identify a functional problem. There must therefore be some transition that occurs in the mind of both the therapist and the patient to focus on the disabilities rather than the impairments. The assessment instruments used by many therapists focus on a description of the impairments. However, the assessment must generally lead to a functional description encompassed by a measure such as the functional independence measure (FIM) or Barthel index (BI). These measures contain items of performance such as dressing, transfer from bed to chair, and ambulating. The status at the outset in each of those areas is determined as well as the long-term goals to be achieved to ensure safe discharge home.

Many rehabilitation programs measure their effectiveness and efficiency by the changes that occur in the patient's status in these performance items between admission and discharge. In some settings, the items themselves are used as a shorthand method to identify the status and goals of the rehabilitation plan. Each FIM item has one to seven levels reflecting degrees of "burden of care." Discussion with the patient can be couched in terms of those numbers. For example, the status on admission on the item reflecting the transfer between bed and chair may be such that the patient is able to carry it out with only a slight amount of physical assistance (scored as 4) with a 1-week goal of being able to perform that task with supervision only needed (scored as 5) and a long-term goal consistent with discharge home to carry out the transfer independent of need for supervision (scored as 6 or 7).

The steps to use in answering each of the questions are also being followed. The exploration of several problems that occurs during the assessment process must lead to a selection of a priority area. To accommodate an enlarged team during the limited time available, each therapist would identify for discussion one single area in which a short-term goal can be brought to the team for discussion. The basis for selection of this priority area can differ. One criterion has been for the selected goal to be one that lends itself to the requirement for coordination for the formation of a **team goal** defined as one requiring at least two of the professional staff to work together. Another criterion would be that the team goal be also one with direct relevance to the likelihood of discharge home.

For example, one common team goal brought forward by the physical therapist would deal with mobility. A goal in this area clearly could make a difference in being able to live at home. Depending on the initial status of the patient, the priority in the mobility area could be a goal relating to the transfer from bed to chair or toilet. Such a goal meets the other criterion in that the transfer activity could go on under the auspices of the several team members. Although the physical therapist could be assigned primary responsibility, all the other professionals would normally have occasion to carry out this task with the patient.

At the team meeting, each therapist would then bring one single area to lead to a short-term goal that would be specified and documented to be evaluated at the following meeting. Another example would be a plan generated under the auspices of the occupational therapist dealing with one or another activities of daily living (ADL). One such sub-plan could deal with problems in eating, an ADL that would be carried out on some days under the auspices of the assigned nurse as well as by the therapist primarily assigned to monitor progress in this area. Similarly, a sub-plan commonly developed under the auspices of the speech therapist would include the ability to communicate basic needs (e.g., toileting) or to signify the presence of pain by a person with communication problems. All the various team members would cooperate in carrying out any such plan recommended by the assigned speech therapist. An overall plan could then commonly contain at least three sub-plans from the several therapists. Additional objectives could be set with the patient by each of the team members to be worked on during the individual therapy sessions. However, to meet the time constraints and the necessity for focus to achieve coordination, one brings to the interdisciplinary meeting only those issues that meet the criteria established.

The status and goals descriptions can reflect many of the items used on the FIM. However, the FIM contains only 18 items. Although it reflects many of the issues of mobility and ADL, it is limited in the area of cognition and communication. It contains no items dealing with such important issues as family participation. It is generally necessary to generate statements of goals and status in aspects of the rehabilitation program that are not encompassed by those items available on the FIM.

Table 4-2 describes the team conference report used to document within each of the major areas the present status reflecting progress, the short-term goal, and what worked. The last aspect could also be

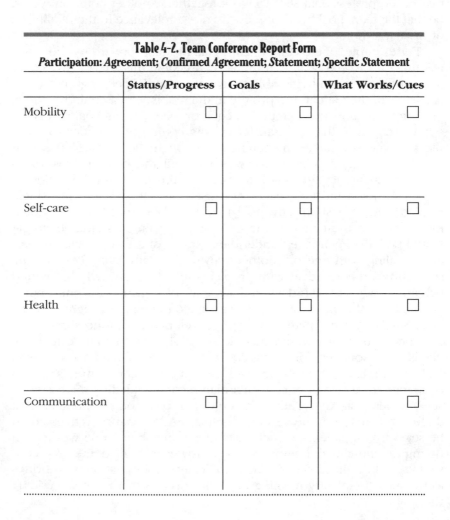

Table 4-2. Team Conference Report Form
Participation: *Agreement; Confirmed Agreement; Statement; Specific Statement*

	Status/Progress	Goals	What Works/Cues
Mobility	☐	☐	☐
Self-care	☐	☐	☐
Health	☐	☐	☐
Communication	☐	☐	☐

described as the cues the therapist might offer to the patient. At the various meetings the appropriate larger boxes would be filled in. For example, at the initial meeting the status and goals could be identified. Table 4-3 illustrates the report for an initial meeting. At subsequent

Table 4-3. Initial Meeting: Team Conference Report Form
Participation: Agreement; Confirmed Agreement; Statement; Specific Statement

	Status/Progress	**Goals**	**What Works/Cues**
Mobility	[A] Transfer mod (50%) assist	[A] Transfer min-mod (35%) assist	☐
Self-care	[A] Dressing upper body mod assist (50%)	[A] Dressing upper body min assist (25%)	☐
Health	[A] Continent of urine during day	[C] Continent of urine (100%)	[A] Calling for bedpan every 3 hours
Communication	[A] Intelligibility 60%	[A] Intelligibility 85%	[A]

meetings, the new status would be documented and what may have worked before now describing a new goal. Table 4-4 illustrates such a subsequent interim meeting. These reports could be duplicated and used by the patient as well as the staff to review the content of the meeting.

Table 4-4. Interim Meeting: Team Conference Report Form Participation:
Agreement; Confirmed Agreement; Statement; Specific Statement

	Status/Progress	Goals	What Works/Cues
Mobility	[C] Transfer min-mod assist (35%)	[C] Transfer min assist (25%)	[A] "Nose over toes"
Self-care	[A] Dressing upper body min assist (25%)	[C] Dressing upper body with supervision	[C] Put into sleeve affected area first
Health	[S] Dry both night and day	[A] Know goal for blood pressure and record results	[A] no fluid at night call for toileting every 3 hours
Communication	[S] Intelligibility 85% with cues	[A] Intelligibility 85% without cues	[C] Take a deep breath

The Patient as Participant

The issue of patient participation in relation to the team meeting can also be dealt with using the principles of the scale described in Chapter 3. The team conference report contains the site where the degree of participation could be documented in relation to each of the questions addressed. The small box within each of the larger boxes is used for this purpose. A notation within this smaller box would indicate that the question was addressed to the patient for consideration as illustrated in Tables 4-3 and 4-4. The actual level of participation achieved would be documented reflecting the scale being used.

The scale in use in this setting is a modification of the one described in Chapter 3. The scale used in the context of the team meeting on a program for persons with stroke is described in Table 4-5. This modified scale reflects the exigencies of working within the time constraints

Table 4-5. Degree of Participation (Stroke)

Patient	Professional
Specific Statement	Asks open question as to *what?*
	Asks for specification
Free Statement	Asks open question as to *what?*
Confirmed Agreement	Asks questions
Puts into his/her own words	Provides recommendation
	Asks for agreement
	Asks for confirmation
Agreement provides assent (or dissent)	Asks question
	Provides recommendation
	Asks for agreement

of the team meeting. Clients were physically present in the team meeting and were addressed in relation to each of the questions. Patients were encouraged to participate at the highest level consistent with the time constraints. Patients with cognitive and receptive language impairments that precluded participation were only a small minority of those normally admitted to an acute rehabilitation program. The percentage would vary with the character of the patients admitted to any such program. Generally, a patient able to consistently signify "yes" or "no" could participate albeit only at the level of "agreement." Problems in expression would limit the ability to participate at the higher levels. If the patient is unable to participate, a family member could serve as a surrogate.

Unlike the policy described in Chapter 3 of starting at the highest participation level and then "moving down" the scale, specific objectives are set for the overall program by the staff for each of the planning sessions. Objectives could relate to the questions to be addressed, the steps in answering those questions (exploration, selection, specification) as well as the level of participation to be sought. Implementation of a program in the management of persons with stroke illustrates the character of the objectives that can be set. At the initial meeting, the objective could be for the patient to address the question as to "status" in one or more priority areas and to seek "agreement" in each instance. Another objective for the initial meeting can be to address the question as to recommended "goal" in the several priority areas at an "agreement" level. The objectives for the next meeting then can be to continue to address the questions as to status and new goal but now to seek participation at better than "agreement" if at all possible. Objectives could also be set in this fashion for subsequent team meetings leading to the incorporation of the question as to "means" as well as status and goal.

One could evaluate the implementation of the efforts at patient participation in relation to two aspects. One deals with the questions, the other with the answers. The question to be addressed, and the number of times it could be addressed during the course of the patient's stay was considered as a measure of implementation. One may recall that an aim is for the patient to eventually ask himself these questions. Each time it was addressed under the auspices of the professional could add to the likelihood that it would eventually be asked independently. In addition, the wording of the questions is designed to impart a message. For example, in addressing the question of problems, the attempt was to make the transition from a focus on impairments to that of functional disabilities. There was the awareness of the possibility of thinking about the future in reference to the question as to goals; of hope by considering the changes in status that occurred when addressing the outcomes question; and then when considering the question as to "What worked?" or "means" there is the possibility of connecting one's actions to the results achieved.

The more a question is brought up for consideration, the more likely it is to be used independently by the patient. Each use of a question could be documented by a notation in the smaller box. The specific notation in that smaller box could then reflect the level of participation actually achieved in respect to answering that question as measured by the scale being used.

The lowest level of participation in Table 4-5 is that of "agreement" to the recommendation made by the professional. This can be described as "forced choice" in that the patient has merely to nod or otherwise indicate assent (or dissent) to the answer provided. The selection step has been carried out by the professional. However, the choice has been made available to the patient for consideration. The principle at work is that there had been an opportunity for the patient to reflect and consider the action before taking it.

The next level of participation rises to that of "confirmed agreement." This marks an important transition because the patients participate to the additional extent of expressing that which they had agreed on albeit already selected by the professional. An even greater degree of internal processing is necessary to enable clients to state what had been agreed on. Importantly, patients have the opportunity to rephrase the answer In the actual verbalization that occurs in the interaction with an attentive listener, patients have a chance to hear for themselves what they are saying.

The next level is that of "statement" reflecting the use of an open-ended question or "free choice." The client has made a selection from the entire universe of possibilities. Once that level has been achieved, the option exists to move the patient to the level of "specified statement." This invites the client to participate at the level of "statement" in answer to the additional open-ended questions as to "How far?" or "How well?" or some other measure of degree. One may note that the 2-point criterion of specificity in this program design sought merely to answer one aspect additional to "What?" rather than the two additional aspects described in Chapter 3.

Several changes were made in the original scale described in Chapter 3. In recognition of the increased difficulties of participation in a group along with problems associated with brain injury and time constraints during the meeting, the order used was to start at the level of "agreement" and then work up the scale as it was possible to do so. Further changes included the use of only three basic categories. These are "agreement," reflecting forced choice, "confirmed agreement" amplifying that which had been chosen, and "statement" reflecting free choice. "Specified statement" merely amplifies the result of the open-ended question. "Multiple choice" was dropped as a category. "No choice" reflecting an order or prescription to which the patient could "go along" in terms of action without previous opportunity to consider was omitted from the scale.

The patient's ability to participate in the team meeting was the aim. It was in that site that evaluation could occur. It was common for each of the therapists to review with the patient at least once before the team meeting their status and what had worked as well as the next short-term goal in preparation for the team meeting. Some therapists found it helpful to do the same on an informal basis at the end of each of the daily therapy sessions.

Alternative formats for measuring patient participation can be designed. These other formats can reflect the type of patient and problems that may occur in encouraging participation in planning. One example is a program designed for inviting the participation of persons with head injury. The scale differs from that developed to deal with persons with stroke. Table 4-6 describes a scale designed for use in an out-

Table 4-6. Participation Scale (Head Injury)

Therapist	Patient
4. Asks open-ended question	Independent statement
3. Makes recommendation/ Seeks agreement/Asks for restatement	Able to restate in own words
2. Makes recommendation/ Seeks agreement	Agrees
1. Prescribes	Willing to go along

patient "transition" program. The questions as to "problem," "status," and "goal" were to be addressed with the client recurrently during the bi-weekly team meetings at which the patient was present. The focus of the meeting was to assess patient agreement to the status of long-term goals leading to discharge. The status of those long-term goals had been discussed previously with the patient by each of the therapists. In the context of the interdisciplinary planning meeting, one could, with the patient present, have his contribution to establishing further priorities particularly as related to discharge. Participation in the team meeting as well as the individual meetings with each of the therapists could improve efficiency because the overall priorities for the team could now be established including such matters as discharge date.

The scale in Table 4-6 incorporates the lowest level of participation ("no choice") from the basic scale format described in Chapter 3. Scale score 1 reflects the willingness to "go along" with the action prescribed by the staff. The patient has no opportunity to participate to the extent of considering the action. It is unlikely that there would be much in the way of commitment of energy to the implementation of any plan generated at this level of participation. Nevertheless, there were instances in this population when because of denial on the part of the patient, documenting that level of participation seemed necessary to the staff designing the program. The next level of participation (scale score 2) reflects agreement to the recommendation made by the professional. Scale score 3 rises to the level of confirmed agreement. The highest level of participation (scale score 4) reflects an independent statement.

The principle remains of the staff being aware of the degree to which patient participation is being sought and has been achieved. By virtue of its ongoing measurement, the likelihood of its achievement is enhanced. The dictum is being followed that, if one expects something to occur, it is usually necessary to inspect for its occurrence.

EVALUATION

Data Collection Intrinsic to Treatment

The principle is that evaluation must be carried out in a timely and cost-effective manner. The model described was carried out by several different teams operating on an in-patient hospital-based program for persons recovering from a recent stroke. The process of data collection was designed to be intrinsic to the clinical setting. Such an approach has major advantages. To meet the constraints of time and cost, the data collection goes on concurrently with the action being evaluated. This serves several purposes. Data collection done immediately obviates the need for later more costly efforts for retrieval of data. The other advantage lies in the opportunity for the person scoring the interaction to be made more aware of the actual level of participation achieved. Given knowledge of the objectives to be met, the greater is the likelihood that one will seek to achieve them. There is immediate feedback of the results to the staff person who is doing the documentation at that time as to the degree to which one is meeting the objective that had been set. Measurement during the team meeting can also contribute to inter-rater reliability of measurement because all persons were present and could simultaneously score the behavior.

The implementation of this process involving the patient or family as a member of the planning team can be evaluated at several levels. The first is the degree to which the total planning process is being implemented in concert with the patient. This is measured by the fact that one or another of the several planning questions have been addressed with the patient. The more often the question is brought to consciousness, the greater the likelihood that the question may arise in the patient's mind independent of it being asked by the professional. Documentation of the question being asked is a notation in the small box in Table 4-2. One could score the total number of times the question was asked.

The wording of the question is important. The wording as to problem transfers focus from the impairments to the functional consequences. Attention paid to the wording of the question as to the goals leads the hearer to consider that one can look to the future. Attention paid to the wording of the question as to status in the review process can lead to an awareness of progress having been made with increased hope for the future. Even more important for a sense of control is the awareness of the import of the question as to the action taken that may have contributed to such progress. The further aim is for the person being asked to consider that the source of such contributions arose from within the patient rather than attributing the effects to outside factors.

The second aspect to be measured is the level of participation actually achieved in answering the questions at any one time or during the course of the patient's stay within the program. The general objective is for the patient to participate at the highest level consistent with meeting the other constraints of efficiency and generating an answer that meets the criteria of specificity. Focus is then on the specific notation made within the smaller box on the team conference report. In the stroke program model being described, the notation would be "A" for agreement, "C" for confirmed agreement, "S" for statement, and "SS" for specific statement. In the format described in use on the program for persons with head injury, a number was used to indicate each of the scale scores.

One can monitor and document various degrees of implementation. Objectives may be limited for any program design and the evaluation process must not overwhelm the constraints of clinical activities. The team leader or other member would be trained in scoring. One can achieve inter-rater reliability by having the team members each score their individual interaction along with the team leader during the team meetings. Each is scoring the same interaction. Ongoing training of staff could continue. The aim is to increase awareness on the part of the entire staff of the level of participation during the team meeting so that the therapists and other staff may then generalize their behavior to other settings. The therapists can then modify their own individual interactions with patients. They can strive to enable an optimal level of patient participation in other settings not under the direct control of the team leader.

One of the constraints in establishing goals for the implementation of the entire set of planning questions was the level of familiarity with those questions on the part of the staff. Staff training occurred in the context of ongoing implementation of the program over a year. During that time, the use of the various questions was expanded in accordance with agreement by the staff. The process by which this was achieved is described in Chapter 5.

Of the several planning questions, the decision was made to offer the patient participation in addressing the question as to goals starting at the initial team meeting. The question as to goal identification had been well established in the lexicon of the therapists in the program dealing with persons with stoke. Therapists were accustomed to setting relatively specific goals with their use of the scale available with the various items in the FIM. The staff was therefore comfortable with offering the patient the opportunity to share in goal setting at the initial team meeting. It was also consistent with the therapist's previous experience to define relatively specific description of status, again with the use of the FIM. There was to be the opportunity for the patient to share in describing status albeit at the second meeting when the initial goals would be reviewed. The implementation of self-conscious patient participation built on the experience in the use of such questions by the staff. The staff was accustomed to make statements of their own in terms of status and goals to which the patients could then agree. The question "What worked?" was generally asked by the staff of themselves less formally and not consistently in the context of team meetings. The staff was not therefore prepared to agree to its use in this first phase of implementation.

Implementation (Phase One)

Table 4-7 describes the limited objectives during the first phase of implementation. The major emphasis was on addressing the questions with the patient rather than the actual level of participation achieved in answering the questions. At the initial team meeting, only the goal question was to be addressed and in three possible problem areas by the appropriate team members. At the interim and discharge meetings, each of the appropriate staff would address with the patient the question of new status in reference to the previously set goal and in the setting of a new short-term goal. Only at the discharge meeting would the question be addressed about what may have contributed to the results achieved. Thus, during a typical in-patient stay encompassing three team meetings, a total of nine opportunities would exist for addressing the goal question, six opportunities for addressing the status question, and one opportunity for addressing the "What works?" question. All three planning questions were to be addressed at the first follow-up ambulatory session in review of the progress made since the time of discharge from in-patient services.

The number of times the question was addressed with the patient can also aid in the ability of the patient to participate in answering the question. The level of participation to be sought thus related to the experience of both the staff and patient functioning at the level of "agreement" as a minimum. Several opportunities to function at the level of "agreement" could then lead to seeking a higher level of participation such as "confirmed agreement." It was felt that one should have a number of opportunities to function at a particular level before seeking to "move up" the scale. The rate with which the therapist could

Table 4-7. Rehabilitation Team Meeting: Patient Participation Objectives Phase 1

Questions Addressed	Initial Team Meeting	Interim Team Meeting	Discharge Team Meeting	Initial Ambulatory Meeting
STATUS/PROGRESS		X3	X3	X3 Confirmed agreement
WHAT WORKED/CUES			X1	X3 Confirmed agreement
GOALS	x3	x3	Confirmed Agreement x3	x3 Confirmed agreement

x = times question addressed with patient; confirmed agreement, patient rephrasing of recommendation made by professional.

move up the scale would of course vary with the individual patient. A general set of objectives, however, had to be set for the several teams and the variety of patients. An initial attempt at setting objectives is reflected in those set in phase one.

The major transition in level of participation was movement from mere "agreement" to some level of verbalization as exemplified by "confirmed agreement." For example, because there were six prior opportunities to address the goal question at the level of "agreement," the objective at the time of the discharge meeting was for an attempt to be made to move beyond that level to seek the level of "confirmed agreement." By the time of the initial ambulatory meeting, there were six prior opportunities to address the question of status at least at the "agreement" level and nine previous opportunities to address the question as to goals. The objective at the time of the initial ambulatory meeting was to seek to reach the level of "confirmed agreement" for both questions. The attempt was also made to address the "What works?" question at a level of greater than mere agreement.

The number of times a question needed to be addressed before adding another question depended on the ease of the staff and the efficiency with which the staff could function during the time-limited team meeting. The experience of the staff working in this model and the facility with which they worked as a team varied. The policy of the administration was to rotate staff among the programs leading to the need for ongoing staff training. For example, a physical therapist may function on the program for persons with stroke for about 6 months before being transferred to working with persons with spinal cord injury. Fortunately, a core of staff remained constant. Another factor requiring ongoing staff development was the application over several teams with somewhat varying styles of the several physicians serving as team leaders. The value of this rotation policy was that staff throughout the various programs began to implement a degree of patient participation in their own individual work. Examples of this more widespread application are described in Chapter 5.

Table 4-8 describes the level of implementation achieved as measured by the number of times a question was addressed during the team meetings. The data analysis procedures had to be kept as simple as possible. It was only necessary for the copies of the team conference report to be reviewed. The presence of a notation in the small box was recorded to be divided by the expected number of occasions for such. The percentage thus reflected the actual number of occasions in relation to the opportunities for such. One may note improvement in the percentages achieved during the course of the two quarters particularly in relation to the status and goal questions. By the second quarter, an

Table 4-8. Level of Implementation Phase One

Questions Addressed	1st Quarter	2nd Quarter
Goal	188/360 or 52%	202/288 or 70%
Status	135/240 or 56%	230/288 or 80%
What Worked	2/40 or 5%	10/32 or 30%

acceptable level had been reached during the in-patient stay. The "What worked?" question was not being addressed throughout the program at the discharge meeting as projected but did show improvement over the two quarters of the year incorporated in this table.

Implementation (Phase Two)

Following the experience during phase one, the acceptance of this new approach by the staff permitted a further level of implementation. Table 4-9 describes the objectives for both the use of the planning questions and the level of patient participation to be achieved in their answers. This second phase incorporated several additional components. On the basis of the level of implementation actually achieved, it became clear that the status question could be appropriately addressed during the initial team meeting in respect to the priority areas. The staff had considerable experience in implementing patient participation in the meeting. It had been shown to be possible. Now the medical and nursing staff had an increased commitment to participation in the program.

Table 4-10 describes the modified plan to be implemented in phase two. There were to be two major plans: a health plan to incorporate prevention of recurrent stroke and the rehabilitation plan dealing with training in methods of community living including the training of family members. The overall number of sub-plans to be dealt with during the team meeting thus might increase with the introduction of health issues requiring even greater attention to time constraints. There was the likelihood of four sub-plans generated and reviewed at each meeting. The schedule for implementation of the health plan by the nursing staff included involvement starting on the day of admission. There was thus an opportunity both to review progress and what worked in respect to the health plan by the time of the initial interdisciplinary team meeting. This meeting would normally occur several days after admission following assessment by the several team members to develop what would be the rehabilitation plan.

Table 4-9. Stroke Recovery Program: Patient Participation Objectives Phase Two

	Day 1	Initial Team	Interim Team	Discharge	Initial Ambulatory
STATUS		*Agreement* Health plan Rehab plans	*Agreement* Health plan Rehab plans	*Confirmed Agreement* Health/Rehab plan	*Statement Level* Health/Rehab plans
WHAT WORKED		*Agreement* Health plan	*Agreement* Health/Rehab plans	*Confirmed Agreement* Health/Rehab plans	*Statement Level* Health/Rehab plans
GOALS	*Agreement* Health plan	*Agreement* Health plans Rehab plans	*Confirmed Agreement* Health/Rehab plans	*Statement Level* Health/Rehab plans	*Specific Statement* Health/Rehab plans

Table 4-10. Stroke Recovery Program: Health/Rehabilitation Patient Self-Management (PSM) Phase Two

	Day 1	Day 2/3 Assessment	Day 3/4 Initial Team	Day 10/11 Interim Team	Day 18/19 Discharge Team	Day 34 I/O Visit
ACTIVITIES	Orientation to PSM Establish PSM (Health) Phase 1	Implement PSM Health plan	Evaluation of Health PSM plan Establish rehab PSM plan	Evaluation PSM health, rehab plans	Evaluation of PSM health, rehab plan	Evaluation of PSM rehab plan
OBJECTIVES	1. Addressed goal 2. Agreement as to goal	1. Address status 2. Agreement as to status and goal	1. Address status, what worked and goal 2. Agreement as to status goal, what worked	1. Address status, process, goals 2. Agreement as to status process 3. Confirmed agreement as to goals	1. Address status, process, goals 2. Confirmed agreement status, process 3. Statement as to goals	1. Address status, process, goals 2. Statement level status and process 3. Specific statement as to process
EVALUATION	1. Checklist in priority health area	1. Checklist in priority health	1. Team conference report	1. Team conference report	1. Team conference report	1. Team conference report

The question regarding goals of the health plan could be addressed on the admission day. All three questions (status, goals, and means) would now be addressed in reference to the health plan during the initial interdisciplinary team meeting and during each of the subsequent meetings. There were thus, during the in-patient stay, opportunity to address the question of status 12 times, to address the question of goals 13 times, and to address the question of means 9 times.

In light of the increased opportunities to address the questions, the level of participation that could be sought would also increase. At the interim meeting, one could seek to enable the patient to speak to goals at higher than agreement level after having had the prior opportunities to address that question at agreement level for at least five occasions. At the discharge meeting, the transition to "statement" level could be sought. In a similar fashion, at the discharge meeting, one could seek to achieve higher than agreement level of participation in respect to the status question after having had the prior opportunities to address that question at the agreement level at least eight times. The aim was to also seek to achieve participation at better than agreement level at the discharge meeting in response to the "What worked?" question after having had the prior opportunity to address that question at the agreement level at least five times. These objectives are but an example of those that may be set. The principle is that one can consider as a basis for setting such objectives in degree of participation in some relationship to the opportunities to address the question at the lower level. The actual objectives set would differ with the character of the patients served and the commitment and the skill of the staff in carrying out the program. Some of the techniques to increase the level of commitment by staff are described in Chapter 5.

Table 4-11 describes the level of implementation actually achieved during the initial quarter of phase two. Two aspects are reviewed. The first is the level of implementation of the questions. There continues to be a satisfactory use of the opportunities available for the use of the questions as to status and goals despite the increase in the opportunities provided. The criterion of 75% utilization of the opportunities for use of the question had been met. The usage for the "What worked?" question continues to be lower than sought. The second aspect of level of participation was reported for the first time. The measure used was the percentage of patients who achieved a level of participation higher than "agreement" at the time of the discharge meeting. The percentage was substantial for both the goal and status questions and about twice that of the means question. These data now are a baseline for further problem-solving with staff to enable an even higher level of participation to be achieved in relation to both aspects of implementation. The

**Table 4-11. Feedback Report
Level of Implementation of Patient Participation
in Team Meetings Phase Two**

Questions Addressed	
Goal	75%
Status/Progress	75%
What Worked/Cues	28%

Level of Participation in Team Meetings

Questions Answered at Confirmed Agreements or Better at Discharge	
Goals	41%
Status/Progress	40%
What Worked/Cues	18%

relatively simple format in Table 4-11 for reporting results enables ongoing timely reports to staff as a basis for ongoing commitment to further implementation.

APPLICATION TO PATIENT CARE II

In this set of exercises there is the opportunity to review and revise our first plan generated with a patient at the end of Chapter 3.

The Review/Revision Process

A patient has been interviewed to develop the initial treatment plan in the exercise at the end of Chapter 3 with the use of the Program Planning Sheet (PPS-1) (see Table 2-3). There is now the opportunity for the review/revision of the initial plan. Evaluation can occur at any time—hourly, daily, weekly, monthly—depending on the patient's condition and the intensity of the treatment program. The first step in the review process consists of exploring any outcomes achieved, particularly in relation to the goals(s) initially set, but not limited to them. Once again, one may select from those that which is the best outcome, which can then be specified. The use of PPS-2 (see Table 3-3) offers the opportunity to carry out this review step incorporating the question as to out-comes along with documentation of the lowest level of participation achieved in relation to the several questions.

For example, a patient interviewed initially identified her problems as follows:

1. I can't lift my right arm.

2. I can't comb my hair with my right arm.

3. I can't wash windows in my apartment.

She selected her concern about combing her hair as her priority. One may note that the first answer was at the level of "impairment" but then was succeeded by statements of a more functional nature.

In setting a goal for her therapy, she eventually specified her goal to be: "I would like to be able to comb my hair with my right hand here in the hospital without having pain in the shoulder." Her lowest level of participation in goal setting was "multiple choice." The time for review was 2 weeks.

At that time, outcomes were as follows:

1. I can comb my hair without pain in my right shoulder.

2. I can reach things in my kitchen cabinets without pain.

3. I can drive my car without pain when going to the store near my house.

The lowest level of participation in answering the question as to out-come was "multiple choice."

In revising her answers as to concerns, she listed the following residual problems:

1. The back of my shoulder still feels tight.

2. I can't move my right arm very fast over my head.

3. I still have some soreness between my shoulder and spine.

She apparently still has some residual impairment although the pain and tightness are no longer interfering with her function. The goal for the future she eventually specified was: "To move my right shoulder as fast as I need when I have to use it to do things, without pain."

PPS-3 (see Table 3-6) provides the opportunity to extend the review process to addressing the question as to "What worked?" to achieve those outcomes before once again revising the plan for the future. This format completes the application to patient care of the entire set of planning questions, once again with attention to the lowest level of par-ticipation achieved. Table 4-12 illustrates the use of the entire set of questions as you might use them with a client.

Table 4-12. Example of Student Use of PPS-3 To Interview a Patient Who Has Been under Treatment for Some Time

Name _____   Date ____8-4-98____

Therapist _____

1. **What results have you achieved?** (List at least 3.) Select your best result with asterisk and have that statement meet the criteria of "specificity."
   A. Walk better
   *B. Get on and off the bed pan in hospital as needed
   C. Turn over better in bed
   Level of participation open-ended questions

2. **What actions did you take that may have helped to bring about those results?** (List at least 3.) Select what you feel was most helpful and meet the criteria of "specificity" for that statement using an asterisk.
   *A. Practiced use of bedpan
      in my room
      each day
      twice a day
      as long as needed
   B. Pulling theraband
   C. Exercises in bed
   Level of participation multiple choice

3. **What problems do you have now? What questions do you have?** (List at least 3.) Select your greatest concern with an asterisk and have that statement meet the criteria of "specificity."
   A. Want to get up and go home
   *B. Need to fix food at home by myself when I get hungry
   C. Can't get things ready for cooking at home
   D. Can't clean up in kitchen at home after cooking
   Level of participation open-ended questions

4. **What would you like to see accomplished which would make you feel that you are making some progress in dealing with your greatest concern?** (List 3.)
   A. To be able to get food together and put it away
   *B. To be able to fix a simple meal for myself at home when hungry
   C. Be able to wash dishes
   Level of participation multiple choice

5. **What is your plan?**
   A. **Goal:** (Please be specific)
      What?   Fix a piece of toast
      Setting?   At home
      To what degree?   Without burning myself

Table 4-12. (Continued)

B. **Means:** (Identify from those actions which may have worked in
2 above)
Exercises in bed to strengthen my arms and hands, using
Theraband, 15–20 minutes a day to the extent that I can depress
the toaster button.
Training in O.T. in kitchen skills
C. **Time Line:** by the end of this month
Level of participation multiple choice

APPLICATION TO PATIENT CARE III

Program Design

In this section, you can carry out the application to your own setting of
the methods used for the design of a program plan as illustrated in this
chapter. It is necessary to define the problems being faced in providing
services to a certain category of patient such as that of stroke, head
injury, or musculo-skeletal problem.

Alternatively, you may need to redesign in-patient or out-patient
services in response to changes in funding. The format for planning on
a programmatic level once again shows the application of the participatory planning process to a variety of situations.

Explore the issues you can identify for your own work or do so
with a planning group. Such a group should be representative of those
who would be expected to take part in the implementation of any program plan that is generated. The problems identified can then define
the goals of what you want to accomplish. Eventually, you will need to
specify those goals so that they can be measured.

As an example, an effort in problem exploration on a program for
persons for spinal cord injury (SCI) identified a clear opportunity to
improve the cost-effectiveness of the rehabilitation process. A major
problem is the frequency of illness in persons with SCI particularly during the first year after discharge from rehabilitation. The efforts to train
patients in managing their health in prevention of infection in the urine
and skin ulcers was not effective. One method to improve results in the
maintenance of health would be to use the approach described in this
book. A health plan would be generated as part of the training process.
That plan would have to be one that the patient would be more likely

to carry out after discharge. It would be necessary to involve the patient to the maximal extent possible in making the plan so that he would be more likely to carry it out because it would be his. The patient could practice carrying out the various steps while under supervision before discharge. It was anticipated that persons with paraplegia would be primarily responsible for carrying out their own health management plan. However, it was important that the family members were also informed so that they could support the effort. The ultimate goal would be the measurement of days lost by illness or costs for hospitalization. Various measures could be used. The evaluation system dealing with the degree of implementation is analogous to that designed to measure the degree of implementation of the stroke program described in this chapter.

Table 4-13 describes the design of the SCI program of the procedures for implementation over the course of the patient's stay coordinated with the recurrent team conferences. The patient would be present at each of the meetings after the first. By the time of discharge, he would be expected to communicate this health plan to his family member as a test of his accomplishment. During a follow-up visit within 1 month after discharge, his health plan would be reviewed. Three areas for health promotion were identified: skin, bowel, and bladder. In each instance, goals were to be identified with the patient; the patient would monitor his status on a log sheet and would be able to review the methods being used to accomplish the goals. The measures of the degree of participation were modified to include the use of written material. For example, the principle of "confirmed agreement" could be met by the client reading aloud to his family member what his plan is.

The implementation of the Health Promotion Plan on the Spinal Cord Injury Program required the design of the forms for data collection. One could use an adaptation of the report form described in Table 4-2. A form was also designed for use in data collection during the follow-up visit entitled the Health Promotion Questionnaire. Data collection and analysis could be carried out analogous to the methods described for the stroke program.

At this point, you have the opportunity to design and put into practice an interdisciplinary coordinated effort to implement the Participatory Planning System. Table 4-14 is the format used for planning of the modules described in this chapter. Note that you can modify the time line on the horizontal axis. In general, the principle is to carry out at least one cycle. That is, after an initial plan is made there is the opportunity for review/revision at least once. It is preferable that there be at least two opportunities for the cycle to be repeated so that there can be increased opportunity to reinforce the concept of recurrent nature of the planning process. The vertical axis of the form contains objectives

Table 4-13. Spinal Cord Injury (SCI) Health Promotion (HP) Module Planning Form

	Initial TC	TC #1 with Patient	Interim TC	D/C Conference	Follow-up Post D/C
Objectives	1. Integrate HP into interdisciplinary plan (IDP). 2. Initiate specific first priority.	1. Review and revise first priority area (skin). 2. Initiate second priority (bladder). 3. Integrate patient into IDP.	1. Review/revise first and second priority areas (skin and bladder). 2. Initiate third priority area (bowel). 3. Increase patient participation.	1. Review/revise all areas. 2. Review/revise caregiver training by patient if tetraplegic.	1. Review/revise all areas.
Activities	1. Identify problem areas with patient caregiver. 2. Identify priority areas (skin, bladder, bowel) and establish mutually agreed on goals.	1. Review goals and status with patient/caregiver. 2. Identify what's working. 3. Develop/revise goals. 4. Initiate caregiver training. 5. SCI education classes begin.	1. Review goals and status with patient/caregiver. 2. Identify what's working. 3. Develop/revise goals. 4. Continue caregiver training. 5. SCI education classes continue until completion.	1. Evaluate caregiver training. 2. Retrain/reinforce skills.	1. Review status of goals with patient/caregiver if tetraplegic. 2. Revise goals.
Evaluation	Team Conference Sheet Nursing data base	Team Conference Sheet	Team Conference Sheet	Team Conference Sheet	Health Promotion Questionnaire

Note: TC, team conference; D/C, discharge conference.

103

Tale 4–I4. Module Planning Form

	Date/Time	Date/Time	Date/Time	Date/Time
OBJECTIVES				
ACTIVITIES				
EVALUATION				
RESOURCES				

and activities, which should be self-evident. The evaluation component refers to the site in which data would be documented. One may recall the principle of having the documentation occur integral to clinical interaction. The resources section is useful for defining the actual staff responsible and their time requirements to establish the costs of the various activities.

Chapter 5

Integration in the Clinical Setting

THE GOALS OF THE CHAPTER

This chapter discusses the incorporation of the patient or family into the clinical planning treatment process in a number of different ways. A range of types of patients and their problems are described to illustrate the wide range of the approach. The examples are also used to illustrate the flexibility of the ways you can use the planning questions and the steps in answering them as well as the level of participation sought. The unifying theme is the maintenance of the principles of carrying out a planning process as the underlying structure while being flexible in its application.

The first aspect of integration in the clinical setting is how to integrate the use of the planning questions into the clinical record. It can be made compatible with the SOAP note and other formats for recording clinical data. The second aspect of integration is implementation of this approach in settings where cost constraints exist. This can include use of treatment groups as one alternative way of reducing costs. The third aspect illustrating clinical applications is how one or another question may be used recurrently. Particular emphasis is placed on the value of patient participation in the design of treatment procedures as a means of increasing the degree of implementation of recommended regimens.

INTEGRATION INTO THE CLINICAL RECORD

The information gathered in the patient interview must be integrated into the clinical record. Table 2-3 (PPS-1), Table 3-3 (PPS-2), and Table 3-6 (PPS-3) are a series of generic forms of increasing complexity based on the procedures described in this book as the Participatory Planning System (PPS). Any of these forms can be used to document the actual interview with the patient. They can contain not only the answers to the planning questions but some measure of the degree of participation achieved in answering them. The actual format required for use in the clinical record can vary.

Therapists in clinical practice are always pressed for time and must make the interview as efficient as possible while still encouraging patient participation. It is important to keep in mind that the aim is merely to maximize patient participation. Therapists encourage patient participation as much as possible within the time constraints. Although it is not necessary to maintain the interaction at a "free choice" level, it is necessary to be aware of when one is moving to a lower level of participation. It is this consciousness that enables the therapist to maximize the degree of participation while not requiring one to reach any predetermined level. If one finds it necessary to move "down the scale," it is with the understanding that any reduction in the level of participation may reduce the degree of patient commitment. The total amount of time cannot increase. Rather the objective can be to use the time available in the most effective way. It is a matter of "working smarter rather than working harder."

As part of the integration of the interview in the clinical record, one can list the level of participation achieved in generating the statements. It is advisable to list the lowest level of participation achieved in answer to any of the questions. For example, in answering the question regarding concerns, if the patient required moving to a "forced choice" in the specification step but dealt with the exploration step on a "free choice" level, the final product described in the clinical record would have documentation of the need for "forced choice." It is the lowest level of participation that would limit the commitment made.

Narrative Notes

Therapists are required to use a number of specific formats. Table 5-1 illustrates the use of data derived from the clinical assessment and the patient interview using PPS-1 (see Table 2-3) as a narrative format for the clinical record. Table 5-2 illustrates a shorter narrative derived directly from the patient interview as documented on PPS-1.

Problem-Oriented Clinical Record

One format for documentation that has received wide acceptance is the Weed system, or the problem-oriented medical record (POMR), which is described in more detail.

The SOAP note is written into the medical record. In the SOAP format, S stands for subjective and traditionally contains the statement of the patient's presenting complaints. O stands for objective findings as a result of observations, tests, and measurements made by the therapist. The A section contains the therapist's assessment or interpretation of the subjective and objective findings. Last, the P portion represents the plan for remediation of impairments and disabilities.

Table 5-1. Patient's Medical Record Using a Narrative System and Incorporating the Contents of PPS-1

HPI: A 56-year-old white female referred for evaluation and treatment by Dr. S. Her chief complaint is pain and stiffness in the right shoulder, especially when doing activities that involve using the RUE above the head. The symptoms have not changed significantly over the last month and began insidiously approximately 4 months ago. The pain is described as an ache which is increased with overhead activities (e.g., combing hair, reaching into cabinets, etc.) and relieved with rest. Patient denies a PMH of a similar problem.

Problem Statements: Patient is concerned that (1) *pain prevents her from combing her hair when it needs it, so that it looks good; (2) she cannot reach into overhead cabinets in her kitchen without discomfort; and (3) she has to ask her husband to help her with housework. Patient was cooperative; concerns were elicited with open-ended questions.

Goals: Patient will be able to comb and arrange her hair to her satisfaction, whenever needed, without pain by the end of 2 weeks. Goals were listed using multiple-choice questions.

Evaluation:
Neck: negative during upper quarter scan (AROM, PROM, accessory motion tests, special tests, and palpation).
AROM R shoulder: abduction 0–100°, flexion 0–120°, external rotation 35°, internal rotation 55°. Patient reports a 4 level pain at end-range flexion and rotations. L shoulder WNL without pain.
PROM R shoulder: abduction 0–110°, flexion 0–130°, external rotation 35°, internal rotation 60°. The chief complaint is reproduced during all motions with end-range PROM. End feel is capsular with flexion, internal rotation, and abduction; external rotation produces a spasm end feel.
Resistive isometric tests: decreased ability to generate tension with abduction, producing pain; all other motions are WNL without pain.
Accessory motion tests: anterior and inferior glide are decreased compared with uninvolved side; all others are WNL; all are without pain.
Palpation: unable to reproduce CC with palpation locally and from all dermatomally related structures.
Posture: no significant postural deviations.

Working hypothesis: Patient is unable to comb hair and reach into cabinets without pain because of inflammation in the area of the supraspinatus tendon, decreased AROM (flexion and external rotation), and decreased anterior and inferior glide of the humerus.

Criteria for testing the hypothesis: No pain with resisted abduction; AROM flexion to 150° and external rotation to 60° without pain; anterior and inferior glide of the humerus equal to uninvolved side.

Treatment strategy:

Treatment specifics:

Table 5-2. Narrative, Problem-Solving Format for Recording of Concerns and Goals

1. Initial Data

    2/4/96. 17-year-old male referred from ER by Dr. Dementia for evaluation and treatment of acute (L) ankle sprain which happened this AM during football practice. X-rays negative, patient to take aspirin QID. PMH unremarkable.

    Patient states he hurt his ankle while being tackled during football practice this morning.

2. Problem Statement and Goals

    Patient is worried about (1) being cut from the team, (2) his leg hurts, and (3) (cc) he can't walk on his LLE. These were elicited by giving multiple-choice options on 1 occasion.

    STG: patient will return to normal activity during sporting events (e.g., running, football) and be pain free.

    LTG: 1. full active and passive ROM in therapy, pain free

           2. weight bearing on LLE when walking, pain free

    Patient verbalized these goals in response to open-ended questions.

There is need for some modification of the usual SOAP note to bring it into conformity with the Participatory Planning System. The data as to concerns or problems can be placed in the S portion of SOAP. However, rather than merely listing the first or presenting complaint, the opportunity exists to list several concerns elicited in the exploration step and then identify the major concern. Alternatively, one may list but one major concern after it has been selected and specified in accordance with the procedures described in Chapter 2.

The data generated for patient goals can be placed in the P portion of the SOAP note. Table 5-3 illustrates the use of the concerns and goals portion of the SOAP note format. Several concerns are explored before selection of the "best" statement as indicated by the asterisk. The goal statements are then explored in relation to the selected concern. The first goal is long range; the selected goal is somewhat less so.

Data elicited in reference to the ongoing evaluation of outcome has not been explicitly dealt with in the Weed system. When this Participatory Planning System approach to planning has been used in conjunction with the SOAP note, therapists in clinical practice have chosen to place data regarding outcome at the start of the note in the S portion because it is subjective in origin. Once again, one may choose to list several statements of outcome that were elicited in the exploration step. Alternatively, one may choose to list only the outcome that has been selected as most important and specified. Along with this information

---

Table 5-3. The Concerns and Goals Portion of a SOAP Note

HPI and PMH

1/14/97. 38-year-old white female referred for evaluation and treatment of an acute (R) knee strain which happened 1/10/97 while the patient was playing tennis. Patient reports hearing a "pop" in the (R) knee after (R) ankle plantarflexed and inverted. Following these events, patient reports falling down. No trauma to ankle. PMH unremarkable.

S:

Patient is worried about
1. Not being able to drive,
2. Falling down and injuring the knee more severely, and
*3. Not being able to play tennis.

P:

Patient Goals
1. Wants knee to be "normal like the way it was before my injury" while she is playing a singles and a doubles to the degree that she can play without pain in the knee.
2. Wants to be able to participate in physical activities with family members in her free time without pain in the (R) knee.
*3. Wants to be able to exercise independently in her free time without pain in the (R) knee.

Concerns were elicited with open-ended questions; goals required multiple choice options on 2 occasions.

---

would be a description of the lowest degree of patient participation in making this statement. Table 5-4 illustrates both an initial SOAP note and a re-evaluation 1 week later using both the S and P portions of the SOAP note format.

It is important to maintain the distinction made in this book between goals and means. The word plan in most clinical settings is understood to describe the activities or actions to be taken. There seems to be no clear provision for documentation of the goals to be achieved by those actions. It is clearly necessary to include both ends and means in any plan. Lack of clarity as to goals or ends would prevent satisfactory review of those goals or any rational selection of means. It has been useful to use the P or plan section of the SOAP note to describe the goals as well as the methods to be used. We have designated the goal as the initial portion of any plan. The goals generated with the patient can be designated as P-1 and contain both short- and long-term

---

Table 5-4. Example of a Progressive SOAP Note with Regard to System of This Manual, Other Content is Omitted

---

7-1-97. Initial evaluation

S: (elicited with open-ended questions)

1. Patient cannot play golf once a week with his friends as he did a year ago because holding a golf club in his hand is painful.
2. Patient cannot spread mayonnaise on bread, open a jar or milk carton when he wants to eat without someone helping him hold the food items.
*3. Patient cannot dress himself without help from his wife.
 * = Chief complaint

P: Goals; elicited with open-ended questions

1. Patient wants to be able to put on his socks by himself.
2. Patients wants to put on his pants by himself.
*3. Patient wants to be able to put on his shirt without help.
 * = Most important goal

7-8-97. Reevaluation

S: Results achieved in relation to previous goals; obtained through open-ended questions

1. Patient can put on shirt by himself in 5–7 minutes.
2. Patient can tie shoes in less than 10 minutes when getting dressed.
3. Patient can button and zip trousers.

New problems: obtained through multiple choice questions

1. Patient cannot hold or swing golf club well enough on the golf course to play 1 hole of golf.
2. Patient does not have enough flexibility to reach down and hold trousers while putting his legs in.
*3. Patient cannot get his hand behind his back when getting dressed to get belt through the belt loops.
 * = Chief complaint

P: Goals; obtained by making recommendations

*1. Get hand in back when getting dressed so he can get belt through belt loop
2. Be able to grasp golf club firmly enough on the golf course so he can practice putting, using his L arm to help guide the club
3. Be able to put his pants on unassisted

Time line: To be accomplished in 6 months

---

goals as needed. One could specify those goals that are of the highest priority. Once again, some statement should describe the degree of patient participation in relation to the goals. The plan will incorporate patient input concerning not only the goal but the time line, which

Table 5-5. Portions of a SOAP Note Illustrating the Incorporation of Data Collected in a PPS-2 Format

Problems: (in the POMR chart, these are found on a separate page)
1. L-3 incomplete paraplegia
2. Burst fx s/.p CRIF with bone graft @ L-2 to L-4
3. R scapular fx
4. R 5th metatarsal fx
5. Fx of L pubic ramus
   achieved using open-ended questions

S: Outcomes:
*1. I can sit in my wheelchair with less pain in my LLE.
2. I can bring myself to sitting at bedside with minimal assistance.
3. I can put my brace on by myself.

What worked:
*1. By closing my eyes and slowing down my breathing for 5 minutes or less, wherever I am, whenever I have pain in my LLE, I can relieve the sharp pain in my LLE.
2. By pulling my LEs up to my chest with my UEs, as far as I can without pain, and by sitting up, I can push myself to the side of the bed.
3. I put the arm rail at the side of the bed to assist me in rolling so that I can put on my brace.

Concerns:
*1. My hamstrings are too tight to allow me to sit at 90° hip flexion.
2. I can't reach my LE with one hand and hold myself in sitting with the other hand without assistance.
3. I can't get my pants on around my ankles without assistance.

Subjective data obtained through multiple choice questions

O: Patient performed transfers w/c < > bed with safety guarding. Patient performed pushups while prone, 10X. Patient is able to come from prone to long sitting with hips flexed at 80°.

A: Patient progressing quite well with treatment. Patient seems to be experiencing much less discomfort during sitting. Patient's rehab. activities are restricted by tight hamstrings. Patient is quite motivated for treatment.

P-1: (goals)
*1. To achieve greater ease in performing bed mobility activities and transfers, to the degree that he can come to 90° of hip flexion
2. Patient wants to be able to bring LEs to the side of the bed independently.
3. Patient wants to put on pants independently.
4. Increase hamstring flexibility
5. Increase LE strength
6. Independent in bed mobility
7. Independent in long sitting and bench sitting
8. Independent in w/c on uneven surfaces

Table 5-5. (Continued)

P-2: (means)

    Continue present treatment, i.e., slow breathing with eyes closed, pulling LEs to chest, pushing to side of bed, practice putting on brace. Begin sitting balance activities, bed mobility activities, and w/c activities on uneven surfaces.

P-3: Time-line: by December 1

    Plans obtained through multiple choice questions.

could be designated as P-2. Patient input into the third aspect or means can be designated as the third component of a plan, P-3.

Table 5-5 illustrates in still another patient the transfer of data generated by this more complete PPS-3 onto the SOAP format. It illustrates how the entire process can be documented in the medical record using the Weed system. Note that any information that comes from the patient's evaluation of the situation is under S, subjective information. This includes concerns, patient's impressions of outcomes, and what worked. If the therapist has other impressions about concerns, outcomes, and what was efficacious in treatment, or the information is based on measured data, it should go under O, observations. It should be under A, assessment, if it is a professional judgment. Goals and plans go under P, plan, separated if necessary into patient goals and therapist goals. For example, in Table 5-5 goals 4 and 5 are therapist goals and reflect a more kinesiologic orientation. Both S and P should contain statements of level of patient participation in arriving at the information recorded there. Also note that under "what worked," each of the three items relates to a different outcome in the section above it. Under P-1 the first three goals relate to each of the three concerns listed above. This can be an acceptable alternative to having "what worked" and "goals" relate only to the most important outcomes or concerns. Note also the flexible use of the format, for example, eight goals instead of three.

Health Care Financing Administration (HCFA)/ Third-Party Payers

In addition to the documentation in the clinical record, payers have a number of requirements for documentation. An example of a widely used one is the requirement by HCFA for documentation of initial, ongoing, and final plans of care. These forms do not stand alone as methods of documentation but are parts of a system that include physician's orders, daily or weekly progress notes, and team conference notes. Data gathered from a PPS can be used to complete sections of the 700 and 701 series of forms. Unfortunately, no provision is made on these forms for documentation of the level of patient participation in answering these questions. Nevertheless, the questions addressed in the PPS are fully compatible with the data normally required for planning for patient treatment.

Table 5-6 illustrates the completion of the appropriate form with data derived from the PPS. The example is that of the 700 form used both initially and at the end of a certification period. Section 20 of the form contains the initial evaluation findings derived from the professional assessment. The patient's concerns as elicited by the PPS, including level of participation, can be entered in this section along with the professional assessment. Section 12 contains both the long- and short-term goals, which can be derived from the PPS along with documentation of level of patient participation. The plan in section 12 can list the means to be used to accomplish the goals. Modalities entered are usually general (e.g., education of the patient/family/caregiver, training in activities of daily living). More specific means derived from the patient interviews can be included in this section. At the end of the certification period or at discharge, the form is completed with an update of the patient's functional level in section 21. Patient's answers to the outcomes and what worked questions, with levels of participation, can be included in section 21.

If it is necessary to recertify a patient for continuing therapy, an updated plan for continued care is illustrated in Table 5-7 (HCFA 701). Updated concerns can be included in section 18 as a status update and justification for further intervention. Section 13 includes any revision of short- and long-term goals. Similarly, revised means can be included in section 13; the revised answers to the outcomes and questions on what worked can be included in section 22 at the end of the billing period.

USE IN GROUPS

The use of groups can be appropriate for a number of different reasons. One is the need to lower costs. It is helpful to consider how the use of PPS can help to maintain quality of outcome in this less costly clinical format. Still another value of the group format is the degree to which sharing can occur among members of the group under the auspices of the professional. The consciousness with which the planning questions are used and their flexibility is one aspect. Still another is the degree to which the group leader has an awareness of the degree to which participation occurs. There is variety in the membership of the groups, in the range of the planning questions to be addressed, and the measurement of the levels of participation achieved.

Group Procedures

The procedures in leading a group are essentially the same as those used with an individual-professional pair. In answering each of the questions, the steps of exploration, selection, and specification can be performed as described in Chapter 2, but now in a group setting. The exploration step follows the model of "brainstorming" in which judgment is deferred. Such deferral of judgment during exploration encourages as much input as possible from the group members. In accordance with the concept of three-fold exploration, the total number of ideas listed by a group of 10 persons could be in the range of 25 to 30.

It is possible even in a very large group for persons to be allowed to speak for themselves. Participants are asked to volunteer their concerns, and efforts are made to encourage as many as possible to participate on a "free" level. No judgment is made as ideas are placed on a chalkboard or easel paper. Neither positive nor negative comments are made. Participants can ask for clarification if the ideas are not understandable, but any statements by the group leader evaluating the ideas tend to reduce the free flow. Only after the exploration step would the opportunity be provided for judgment in the selection step. After many have spoke freely, others who had not participated can be asked. This gives them the opportunity to confirm their agreement to some of the other ideas already listed. To meet the criterion for this level of participation, participants are asked to put into their own words the statements they agree with. It is important to enable such persons to state their own version of the ideas they have agreed on. It has been our experience that each person's ideas differ somewhat in detail. A still lower level of participation could be merely stating their agreement to one or another statement on the list without being verbalized by the participant.

The data derived from a large group during the exploration step generally need to be reduced to be manageable enough to be used in the subsequent steps. Reduction to three to five ideas is generally necessary. The various ideas can be collated so that the group can then carry out the selection step together. This collation process is important. It can be done by the group leader together with some representatives of the overall planning group. An alternative is to use the group to carry out this "clustering" step preparatory to the selection step when

Table 5-6

PLAN OF TREATMENT FOR OUTPATIENT REHABILITATION (*COMPLETE FOR INITIAL CLAIMS ONLY*)

1. PATIENT'S LAST NAME	FIRST NAME M.I.	2. PROVIDER NO.	3. HICN

4. PROVIDER NAME	5. MEDICAL RECORD NO. (*Optional*)	6. ONSET DATE	7. SOC. DATE

8. Type: ☐ PT ☒ OT ☐ SLP ☐ CR ☐ RT ☐ PS ☐ SN ☐ SW	9. PRIMARY DIAGNOSIS (*Pertinent Medical D.X.*) Ⓑ L/E amputee	10. TREATMENT DIAGNOSIS Ⓑ L/E amputee	11. VISITS FROM SOC.

12. PLAN OF TREATMENT FUNCTIONAL GOALS

GOALS (*Short Term*) In 2 weeks, pt. will: 1) Cook breakfast in rehab. kitchen to include turning on/off burner, frying egg & fixing a piece of toast while in wheelchair using adaptive equipment c̄ min Ⓐ

PLAN (*Means or methods*)
–ADL training
–Functional mobility training
–Adaptive equipment training
–V/E modalities
–Positioning/adaptations

OUTCOME (*Long Term*) Return home using a wheel-chair for mobility, adaptive equipment PRN & no greater than min Ⓐ from family &/or aides.

13. SIGNATURE (*professional establishing POC including prof. designation*)	14. FREQ/DURATION (*e.g., 3/Wk x 4 Wk.*)

I CERTIFY THE NEED FOR THESE SERVICES FURNISHED UNDER
THIS PLAN OF TREATMENT AND WHILE UNDER MY CARE ☐ N/A

15. PHYSICIAN SIGNATURE | 16. DATE

20. INITIAL ASSESSMENT (History, medical complications.
Level of function at start of care. Reason for referral)

Pt. stated her 3 concerns are: 1.) transferring from bed to wheelchair to bedside
commode, *2.) cooking while using her wheelchair, & 3.) giving herself a bath
(free choice for all 3 responses)

* Greatest concern

21. FUNCTIONAL LEVEL (End of billing period) Progress Report   ☒ CONTINUE SERVICES OR ☐ DC SERVICES

Pt. was an active participant in OT this billing period and requires continuing
skilled services. Goal status is as follows: STG1 – Cook breakfast in rehab–addressed,
achieved, goal will be upgraded to supervision level. She found using *long handled
reacher to turn stove controls, a lap board on her W/C to carry items, & pre-planning
the activity to be helpful (*most helpful).

17. CERTIFICATION

FROM   THROUGH   ☐ N/A

18. ON FILE (Print/type physician's name)

☐

19. PRIOR HOSPITALIZATION

FROM   TO   ☐ N/A

22. SERVICE DATES

FROM   THROUGH

Table 5-7

DEPARTMENT OF HEALTH AND HUMAN SERVICES
HEALTH CARE FINANCING ADMINISTRATION

☐ Part A   ☐ Part B   ☐ Other _____ Specify

UPDATED PLAN OF PROGRESS FOR OUTPATIENT REHABILITATION
(Complete for Interim to Discharge Claims. Photocopy of HCFA-700 or 701 is required)

1. PATIENT'S LAST NAME	FIRST NAME	M.I.	2. PROVIDER NO.	3. HICN

4. PROVIDER NAME	5. MEDICAL RECORD NO. (Optional)	6. ONSET DATE	7. SOC. DATE

8. Type: ☐ PT ☒ OT ☐ SLP ☐ CR ☐ RT ☐ PS ☐ SN ☐ SW	9. PRIMARY DIAGNOSIS (Pertinent Medical D.X.) Ⓑ L/E amputee	10. TREATMENT DIAGNOSIS Ⓑ L/E amputee	11. VISITS FROM SOC.

12. FREQ/DURATION (e.g., 3/Wk x 4 Wk.)

13. CURRENT PLAN UPDATE, FUNCTIONAL GOALS	PLAN (Means or methods)
(Specify changes to goals and plan) GOALS (Short Term) In 2 weeks, pt. will: 1) Cook a typical meal in rehab. kitchen while in wheelchair using adaptive equipment PRN c̄ supervision. OUTCOME (Long Term) Return home using a wheelchair for mobility, adaptive equipment PRN & no greater than min Ⓐ from family &/or aides.	–ADL training –Functional Mobility Training –Adaptive Equipment Training –V/E Modalities –Positioning/adaptations

I HAVE REVIEWED THIS PLAN OF TREATMENT AND
RECERTIFY A CONTINUING NEED FOR SERVICES. ☐ N/A ☐ DC

14. RECERTIFICATION

FROM   THROUGH   ☐ N/A

15. PHYSICIAN'S SIGNATURE   16. DATE

17. ON FILE (Print/type physician's name)   ☐

18. REASON(S) FOR CONTINUING TREATMENT THIS BILLING PERIOD
(Clarify goals and necessity for continued skilled care)

Pt. still requires skilled OT services to address short term goals leading to long term goal
of returning home. She achieved STG of cooking breakfast in rehab. kitchen using W/C & adaptive equipment c̄ min Ⓐ & goal has been upgraded to supervision only. The 3 concerns about
cooking with less physical Ⓐ are: 1.) reaching heavy, hot items, 2.) carrying heavy, hot
items from one area to another, & *3.) maneuvering w/c safely c̄ injuring her stumps.

* Greatest concern

19. SIGNATURE (or name of professional,
including prof. designation)   20. DATE   21.

22. FUNCTIONAL LEVEL (at end of billing period—Relate your documentation to functional outcomes and list problems still present)

☐ CONTINUE SERVICES or ☐ DC SERVICES

23. SERVICE DATES

FROM   THROUGH

priorities will be assigned. Doing so enables the building of consensus as one establishes priorities. One method has been to form subgroups of three to five persons who then "cluster" the various ideas listed by the large group. The instruction to each of these smaller groups is to list three categories that would encompass all the ideas listed by the entire group in the exploration step. Each cluster would retain the ideas subsumed, thus characterizing the cluster in detail. This clustering procedure permits the retention of the original variety of ideas but in a more manageable way. The important group consensus can come about by finding similarities among the clusters developed by each of the small groups. It is common for considerable similarity to be found in the clusters generated by each of the small groups. Generally there are but three to four clusters that can be agreed on. One can then specify those several clusters agreed to be in common or even one that is considered to be of the highest priority.

The actual selection step can be handled in various ways. The aim is to establish priorities to allocate resources effectively. Another format for working from a large list generated during the exploration step is to have individual group members select three important concerns from those generated by the entire group. Those items with the largest number of votes can then be assigned weights. A shared weighting procedure as described in Chapter 2 is used to determine the priorities for each of the persons in the group who can then make a commitment for their own subsequent plans.

Program Planning Group

WHAT IS THE PROBLEM? There is need to make clinical services more cost effective. In addition to the lowering of costs, the opportunity lies in improving outcomes. One method for doing so is to enlist the energy and the ideas of those who are unpaid, that is, the patients. The implementation of the PPS within any clinical setting requires a change in the focus of the work with patients. The PPS planning format can be used with a group of professionals to generate a plan for the design of a training program for implementation of the PPS in patient care. It is desirable for any such change to come about with the contribution of the energy and the ideas of the staff. The aim is to enlist such energy and commitment by involving the staff in the design of the changes. One works with the staff in the format consistent with the format they will be using with their clients.

THE PLANNING PROCESS. The first question is asked about the problems and concerns of the staff. Table 5-8 is a large list of concerns elicited from a therapy staff group; 20 items were generated. Table 5-9 illus-

---

Table 5-8. In-Service, Session 1

Exploration of group concerns of involving patients in program planning
   1. Cognitive status, concerns pre vs post injury
   2. How much can they be involved; abstraction; short-term and long-term carry-over after discharge
   3. Follow-through after discharge
   4. Depression and denial interferes with motivation to accomplish goals
   5. If patient denies, will he plan treatment
   6. If patient included, therapist not doing job
   7. Patient fear of interacting with professionals
   8. Overachievers may set unrealistic goals
   9. Newly disabled—long time to realize what goals are possible
  10. For old disabled—long time to realize what goals are possible
  11. Professionals would have to change attitude toward patient
  12. What if patient's goal doesn't correspond with M.D.'s goal?
  13. With children, goal setting and communication with family is a problem
  14. Difficult setting goals with changing status—deteriorating or improving
  15. Overburdening parents with therapy responsibility
  16. Involving those in goal setting who want to be left alone
  17. Time elements and relationship—takes time to achieve, especially in acute care
  18. Find out the reason they're unmotivated (e.g., pain, failure)
  19. Is it realistic that patient and therapist do all goal setting without M.D.
  20. Financial obligations keep patients from setting goals and attending therapy

---

trates how those items were clustered with retention of the original ideas. Common themes among the concerns were identified. Specific comments that support each major category are included along with the overall theme of the category. Once some value or priority is assigned, one can then explore the question as to goals in the selected high priority area(s) in a similar fashion before specifying the objectives.

Table 5-10 (PPS-1G), a modified version of PPS-1 (see Table 2-3), can be used with groups. It helps organize a group's concerns, their major concerns via clustering, and exploration of general goals. The selected goals can then meet the criteria for specification. A time line for implementation can be generated. The plan has been developed in the context of having explored the staff's concerns and having achieved some commitment in terms of priorities.

Table 5-9. Clustering of Data from Exploration of Concerns in Table 5-8

Realistic goals: Overachievers set unrealistic goals; newly disabled may not realize what is possible; old disabled may require long time to realize what goals are possible; if patient denies, will he plan treatment?

Cognitively impaired: Cognitive status, concerns pre vs post injury; how much can they be involved, abstraction, short-term and long-term carry-over after discharge?

Motivation: Follow-through after discharge; depression and denial interfere with motivation to accomplish goals; find out the reason they're unmotivated (e.g., pain, failure); involving those in goal setting who want to be left alone

Patient, family, and professional relationships: If patient included, therapist not doing job; patient fear of interacting with professionals; professionals would have to change attitude toward patient; what if patient's goal doesn't correspond with M.D.'s goal; with children, goal setting and communication with family is a problem; overburdening parents with therapy responsibility; time elements and relationship—takes time to achieve, especially in acute care; is it realistic that patient and therapist do all goal setting without M.D.?

Skin Ulcer Planning Group

WHAT IS THE PROBLEM? One of the major concerns in the management of persons with spinal cord injury (SCI) is the need for hospitalization for relatively long periods for the treatment of skin ulcers. For example, the SCI service at one hospital had an entire 40-bed unit filled at all times devoted to the treatment of persons with skin ulcers. It was common for patients to seek entry to the hospital with extensive and deep sores leading to lengthy hospital stays, the use of special costly beds, and eventual surgical treatment. The rate of recidivism was high. Patients would leave the hospital after such major treatment only to return within a relatively short time. Opportunities for effective surgical treatments were eventually exhausted due to extensive scarring. The major methods of early treatment and prevention depend on the independent initiative of the person with SCI. The need is to relieve pressure on the skin while lying or sitting. A deliberate set of pressure-relieving procedures must occur in the absence of normal sensation serving as a cue. If a skin ulcer did occur, the treatment again was pressure relief. The aim of the staff was to reduce the frequency of skin ulceration and, if ulceration did occur, to have patients come to the hospital with less severe involvement, thus enabling shorter lengths of stay. The plan was

---

Table 5-10. PPS-16

1. What are the group's concerns (identify average of 2–3 for each partici-
   pant)?
   A.
   B.
   C.
   •
   •
   Z.

2. What are the group's major concerns? Identify 3–4 major themes from
   the list of group concerns and list relevant concerns after each theme
   (clustering). Have group select by either ranking or by weighting.
   Value　A.　Theme _____:
   　　　　 B.　Theme _____:
   　　　　 C.　Theme _____:
   　　　　 D.　Theme _____:

3. What does the group want to see happen? What would indicate to the
   group that it's making progress with the top ranked or weighted cluster?
   Explore and list.
   A.
   B.
   •
   •
   Z.

G, group.

to use the PPS as a method for increasing patient commitment for each
to an individual plan to reduce overall length of stay.

THE PLANNING PROCESS. A "skin care group" was organized in which persons hospitalized with skin ulcers were invited to participate. Three 45-
minute sessions were carried out during the several week length of stay.
The exploration step was used in addressing each of the planning questions to be used. The first session dealt with developing a sense of alternatives in dealing with this problem. Because the topic being addressed
was that of prevention of skin ulcers, the question as to problem was
phrased "What are some of the causes of skin breakdown?". The question was posed on the easel board by the staff group leader. Exploration
was performed by the group answering the question freely on their
own. The staff did not offer ideas unless none were forthcoming. It was
rarely necessary to intervene because each of the persons had problems

with skin breakdown and could deal with his or her own experiences as to what might cause such problems. The staff leader was responsible for encouraging input from all members of the group, with no judgment made as to whether ideas were good or bad. Each idea was recognized by having it placed on the easel board, thus giving evidence of its having been heard. It was thus also possible for the person stating the idea to be certain that it was being heard properly. During the exploration step at least 10 to 15 statements would surface in a group of five to seven patients. Once the exploration step ended, the selection step was carried out by the group to identify the three most important causes or problems. A voting procedure was used wherein each of the members identified what he or she thought was the most important cause. The causes getting the most votes were then used for the next phase.

For each of the problems so identified, the question was then asked "What would work to deal with this problem?" During the exploration step of addressing this question, three solutions were again elicited in reference to each. Because the aim was to enable the patients to consider alternatives, the threefold exploration was important. For example, one of the causes mentioned for skin breakdown was "sitting too long." The solutions generated were "remembering to shift weight," "lifting up," and "paying attention to a burning feeling." If fewer than three possible solutions arose freely from the group, the professional serving as facilitator would offer several choices from the ideas mentioned by other patients in the past. However, the ideas were not listed on the easel board unless spoken by one of the members of the group.

Still other sessions in this same format of encouraging patients to speak for themselves dealt with other aspects that could lead to a reduction in the severity and frequency of pressure ulcers. For example, a second session dealt with the monitoring process and the early identification of skin breakdown if it did occur. The question as to concerns was now phrased "How would you know you had a pressure sore?". For example, the several answers to what was looked for was "redness," "softening of the skin," "hard spot," and "drying." Following this, the question was posed as to what could one do if one did identify a problem. One of the issues that surfaced was how difficult it could be to act to reduce pressure by limiting the time one sat. One man, for example, lived alone and needed to unlock his door for his Meals on Wheels delivery. He was concerned about leaving his door unlocked. Some of the other members of the group offered him some alternatives. The members of the group had begun to ask themselves the question "What works?". The third session in this series dealt with making a plan for themselves. All members could set their own goals in dealing with their problem of skin ulcers and list ideas that they had heard about to help them to reach their goals.

At the end of each session and at the end of the series, the members evaluated the activities just completed. The questions were "What happened in the groups?" and "What results occurred?". After having elicited several outcomes, the question "What did you do that helped to bring about those results?" was asked. From this evaluation came ideas on methods to improve and expand the sessions. An example of the answers on outcome were such statements as "I learned something new that I could use." Among the ideas listed in answer to what worked, the members of the group made such statements as "getting help from others" and "hearing what other people know." The ideas were of course not new. What was new for these men who were noted for recidivism, severity of the sores, and long stays in hospital was the opportunity for those with the problem to be the ones speaking about it. Not only were they speaking about their problems, but they also could take part in considering their solutions and have a role in evaluating what was being done in the sessions.

The effects of these sessions were evaluated in terms of reduced incidence of skin breakdown in these persons. Significant changes occurred in the frequency and severity of skin ulcers in these patients over the next year with consequent reduction in the number of days they were hospitalized. In reviewing with those patients some months later the methods that may have contributed to these changes, many of their comments related to the content of the sessions and the ideas that they heard about what worked. Several patients also specified the ways that the sessions had been conducted as useful. For example, one aspect mentioned was the fact that they were asked to look at different answers to the question and not just one. One man described it as follows: "We had a chance to get different perspectives. There was no right or wrong answer, but we had a chance to think about things." He continued that he used this approach in relation to many other problems he had in dealing with his life since he had learned how to think about his skin problem.

Stroke Prevention Group

WHAT IS THE PROBLEM? Persons with stroke are candidates for recurrent stroke. The same risk factors associated with the person having an initial stroke can cause another one. The effects of a second stroke superimposed on the effects of the first can be much more severe. For example, persons who are able to care for themselves after the first stroke and go home will be far less likely to be able to do so if another stroke were to occur. The risk factors associated with stroke are well known. Some of the better known are associated with control of blood pressure, diabetes, use of tobacco, and cholesterol level. Although the treatment of these risk factors can be identified and prescribed, life-style changes are frequently necessary along with use of medication. The problem is patient follow-through with the appropriate treatments. Sometimes major changes in life-style also require an ongoing commitment. The plan is to use the PPS as a method for increasing patient commitment to making such changes by being asked to address the planning questions. The use of a group was considered because almost all those on an in-patient stroke program had one of these risk factors so that they could share. Each was also being asked to make an individual health plan.

THE PLANNING PROCESS. This group met on a weekly basis. New persons entered the group each week. It was thus necessary to have the group address new concerns depending on the needs of the members each week. The question "What are your concerns?" was asked. Several issues were offered for consideration such as dealing with health, emotional, and interpersonal problems. Persons would volunteer their concerns from the multiple choices. Even persons with language difficulty could participate. They had merely to be able to nod their agreement or disagreement. Opinions as to what was to be selected were elicited without any evaluation by the group leader. The aim was to engender participation. Once an issue was decided on by consensus, the question "What works?" was asked. All were asked to contribute ideas with the objective of at least several alternatives. The other members of the group could offer ideas. Persons who had the problem could then use the ideas to make their own plan including any goals they wished to consider. The following week, the persons who may have been present in both meetings were asked to review the plans they had made and the results as well as the activities they had carried out. These strategies were thus available for use by other members of the group.

Some of the outcomes from the group itself included validation of each person offering ideas, serving as a mentor. There was improvement in the sense of isolation. Each was not alone in having these problems. Relationships were established that continued in other settings. By the group leader attending to maximizing the level of participation, the process enabled the persons to have a sense of control over their situation.

These several instances of application of the PPS to the group setting are but examples of the different sorts of patients with whom this approach can be applied. The questions addressed with the groups were similar to those used in one-on-one situations. The phrasing of the questions as to concerns could vary, but the structure of asking that question remained basic to the remainder of the planning process. In the context of concerns, one could then address one or another of the planning questions. The "What works?" question is particularly versatile. The exploration step was used on a free level in both the staff planning and SCI groups. In working with persons with stroke, the group leader elected to provide a list of ideas from which the group was to select.

INTEGRATION OF THE PATIENT AS THE DESIGNER

The theme of this entire book has been how therapists can improve the design of treatment and make it more effective by enlisting the ideas of those persons most affected. Their contribution of ideas can also lead to greater commitment of energy to the accomplishment of any activity. This concept seems so elementary that most professionals feel that they are indeed doing so. Yet it is useful to do so with greater consciousness.

Case of the Bedridden Man

The following vignette describing a short interaction by a student therapist beginning to apply the principles illustrates the simplicity and value of the approach.

> I was assigned to work with an elderly man who was lying in bed with restraints on both wrists and with side rails up. He was lying flat on his back when I came in. His speech was slurred and somewhat hoarse. He seemed to be emotionally labile. He was tearful and would start to cry as he spoke in answer to any of my questions. I knew he had been seen by another therapist. I had been told that she felt he was too confused for her to work with him. I wasn't sure how to start. I asked him what was troubling him since that was the first question I had been taught to ask. He first pointed to his restraints and tried to pull them off. I asked him if he wanted them off and he nodded "yes." I took them off and followed with the question as to what else he wanted to do. He said "I want to go home." Then following my training, I tried to help him tell me some other short-term goals.

THERAPIST: What do you need to be able to do to go home?
PATIENT: Get up.
THERAPIST: Anything else?
PATIENT: Walk.
THERAPIST: OK, let me help you get up. [The patient assisted me in getting him to a sitting position on the edge of the bed. He sat there for about a minute with his feet close to the floor.]
THERAPIST: Are you ready to walk?
PATIENT: [Nods yes]
THERAPIST: How far do you feel you can walk just now? [When he did not respond for several seconds, I said] Let me offer you some suggestions: Would you like to walk 2 feet, 5 feet, or 10 feet?
PATIENT: 5 feet.
THERAPIST: OK, let's try to walk the 5 feet. [Patient walks in a shuffling fashion, one foot after the other with support from the therapist the 5 feet to the other bed in the room.]
THERAPIST: That was well done. You walked 5 feet as you wanted. Are you willing to walk any further?
PATIENT: No. [I helped him back to his bed helped him to lie down.]
THERAPIST: You accomplished 5 feet to walk from the bed and 5 feet back. What helped you to do that?
PATIENT: [Points to me and starts to cry but then stops himself.]
THERAPIST: I was glad to help. Is there anyone else or anything else that helped you walk? Let me give you some suggestions. It was you telling me what you wanted. It was you moving your feet. It was you telling me how far you wanted to walk. Any of those things that you did that helped?
PATIENT: Me telling you what I wanted.
THERAPIST: It helped you to tell me what you wanted. Tomorrow when I come back to work with you again, I'd like you to tell me what you want to do and we will try to do it together to get you home.

This short vignette illustrates the value of incorporating the planning questions and the opportunities they offer in the context of everyday clinical situations. In re-establishing a sense of control over his life and his body, the therapist has enabled him to gain his sense of integrity as a person. It is the recognition of his right to make contributions by the asking of questions and the recognition of the contributions he has made that can help to bring about the healing necessary for him to once again be independent.

Case of the Man with "Spasms"

Failure to take the medication prescribed or to follow through with a treatment program or to use the equipment designed to help can arise from the lack of "fit" of the actions to be carried out. The timing of the treatments, their frequency, or their complexity can make it more or less likely that the treatments will be followed. The equipment may be too small, too large, or in some way inappropriate. If the review process explores what may have helped in a nonjudgmental way, the opportunity exists for the patient to participate in increasing the "fit" of the procedures by proving information as to what specific aspects of the actions originally recommended were carried out. If the interaction permits the patient a wide latitude for making free contributions, there is a greater likelihood that the patient will describe modifications of the original recommendations that the person made on his or her own. For example, although the original recommendations may have been to wear a hand splint for an hour several times each day but the patient reports that she actually applied it for longer without any discomfort and with good results, the new plan for the future can now include recognition of the procedures or means that were actually effective. The aim is to validate the person as a participant in the design of treatment.

Occasionally, the patient will describe some new idea that seemed to work. One example is that of a man with paraplegia due to SCI with "spasms" of his body that interfered with his ability to push his wheelchair and go outdoors. In reviewing his progress in dealing with his goal of reducing spasms due to pain, he reported some improvement. He attributed the improvement to the stretching exercises that had been recommended. However, rather than stretching with a heavy weight less often, he found that he felt better when he did stretching with lesser weights but more often. He had begun to be more aware of his goals and was measuring the responses in his body as a criterion rather than following some predetermined set of recommendations. When asked about what else may have been helpful, he also mentioned that he had started using ice in the area of pain in his back. He would apply it soon after he began to feel pain after sitting up for long periods. The use of ice became part of his program. He had heard about its use but had not applied it consistently early with the onset of pain. His regimen had been made to "fit" him. The stretching and ice had been made more effective by his involvement in the design of the timing of its use by using the signals from his body.

Case of the Woman with Stroke

The value of integrating instructions offered by the therapist is illustrated in still another case. A woman with a recent stroke had major difficulty in maintaining balance. She had particular difficulty in maintaining anterior-posterior balance, which interfered with her goal of transferring safely from bed to wheelchair. Her impairments were related to her absence of sensation as to where she was putting her feet, complicated with "neglect" of her left side. The therapist felt it unlikely, given experience with a large number of patients, that this lady would be able to overcome her problems so that she could go home. She had difficulty organizing the sequence of necessary movements. The therapist gave her the instructions of using a numbering system for the sequence of activities. It worked somewhat but worked even better when it was the patient telling herself aloud: "1 scoot forward, 2 rock, 3 get up." In making it her own instructions, she changed the wording somewhat. Even more important, in the process of giving herself the instruction she controlled the timing and made it synchronous with her action. She had made it "fit."

Case of the Man with Tetraplegia

The application of this approach to the design of adaptive equipment can make the frequently costly equipment far more likely to meet the needs of the patient. The following example drawn for the design of an appropriate wheelchair can illustrate the value of patient participation. This 35-year-old man had a recent SCI with a neurologic level at C6. During the early postinjury phase, the user described a number of goals or criteria for evaluation of a wheelchair that would fit his needs. One goal was to be able to balance himself while sitting so that he would still be able to use both his arms in carrying out tasks without needing to hook one arm over the back of the chair to balance himself. Another criterion he felt was important was to remove his armrests easily because of his lack of finger dexterity. Still another more personal goal dealt with his life plans to travel widely as he had before his injury. He therefore wanted a wheelchair that could be easily taken apart and stored in a relatively small space. Another high priority for this person, who also happened to be diabetic, was to be able to maintain his physical health and endurance.

In selecting the means for meetings these goals, the patient had the opportunity, on his request, to use a lightweight wheelchair with a variety of levels of back support. He learned that he could counterbalance his weight by leaning rather farther back and thus have both arms free to perform other tasks. When he had been recommended a chair with a high back more consistent with the usual method of dealing with problems in balance, he found himself unable to use the weight of his trunk to counterbalance. He needed to use one of his arms to steady himself. His experience enabled him to contribute to the design process the value of a back support lower than ordinarily recommended. In this instance, as in others in which design issues arise, the principle is not just the particular back height that was selected eventually. The principle is that all the design factors may vary depending on the individual user and his or her characteristics and priorities. For other patients with differing needs, the higher back support may indeed be appropriate.

The selection of what might be other appropriate means for meeting his several goals was aided by a magazine article listing several alternatives available in lightweight wheelchairs. "I knew what the options were myself. I had a chance to think things through for myself before finally selecting the parts I needed." These options included a freely movable rotating armrest and a chair that could be modified for exercise and easily broken down for storage. His several criteria were actually going to be able to be met.

At the time of review several months after discharge, this patient described his wheelchair as meeting his needs well. He had been able to take several airplane trips; balance had not been a problem; and he had been able to participate in wheelchair slalom racing regularly. An initial concern of the staff was that his lightweight wheelchair would interfere with ability to carry out transfers without a transfer board had not turned out to be a problem.

The issue is not the particular components that this person helped select. No single wheelchair is appropriate for everyone, even given the same level of injury. What is significant is the methodology by which the appropriate wheelchair components can be selected, with particular emphasis on the degree user participation was permitted. This user functioned at the level of "free choice" in respect to setting the criteria and at the level of "multiple choice" in selecting the means for meeting those goals by having available to him the options to review. This user probably also functioned at a much higher level of participation than most are able to achieve. The important principle is that he was given the maximal opportunity to participate rather than focus on the level of participation that was actually achieved. One may find far more contributions to be made and more effective use of technology and treatments when the opportunities are made available.

Case of the Woman Runner

Still another case is that of a young woman long distance runner who was no longer able to run without pain in her knee and hip. Pain affected her gait at all times, even in walking short distances at work. Her muscle tightness affected her strength and her endurance. A stretching regimen was recommended as the first stage leading to her eventual goal of being able to run in a 5K race once again. She was given instructions and handouts describing the exercises she was to do. The first set of goals to which she agreed was to be "independent in the use of her stretching program." In review of progress a week later, she and the therapist noted less tenderness and a change in the texture of the tissue in the affected area. In review of what worked, she described the modified regimen she had been following. She showed the therapist the instruction sheet she had made for herself. Her modifications included giving the exercises more descriptive names. For example, she called the "adductor stretch" a "frog stretch." She renamed the "iliotibial band stretch" as "twist and lean stretch." She also rearranged the order of the exercises. She redrew the figures on the handout by making stick figures for herself. In these several ways, she had made the regimen hers. Attentive listening by the therapist to her modifications taught the therapist about how she could make the handout more useful to others. Moreover, it helped the therapist become more aware of the possible value of offering the option to subsequent patients to make a regimen theirs. She could deliberately offer them the option of modifying the regimen in the several ways this patient had done to her apparent benefit. It is the process of making it fit that makes it work. It is the offer of potential ownership that may be worthwhile.

This principle of encouraging the patient to "tinker" with the regimen and make it more nearly one's own seems to be useful across a variety of problems. It is particularly useful with people who have been discouraged by results before. One therapist who used it found her patients "waking up." She could see the patient "liven up, making a commitment of energy." She would encourage her patients to report back any modifications they had made on the first visit after putting any regimen into effect. She had always suggested to patients that they incorporate any exercise program into their daily activities. But now, she found herself actually documenting such efforts and saw them as particularly worth encouraging. For example, one woman working on balance reported on using the recommended exercise when curling her hair or brushing her teeth. Another woman with ankle sprain used the opportunity of taking the dishes out of the dishwasher and putting them away in the cupboard to do the heel raises that had been recommended. By the patients so doing, the therapist could see the possibility of making whatever was done more "integral," more likely to be carried over into ongoing function rather than merely being done in a disjointed fashion. One person reported on her difficulty in carrying out the hamstring stretching as it had been demonstrated. She "played" with it and demonstrated how she had modified it. The therapist felt she could accept the way it was being done. Although it was "not right," it was actually OK and it was "right" for that patient. Indeed what may have made it right for that patient was not only what she had figured out to do but the very fact that she had made it hers by tinkering with it.

APPLICATION TO PATIENT CARE IV

The exercise at the end of Chapter 4 provided the opportunity for the design of PPS at a programmatic level. There is the need for review and revision of any programmatic design. The procedures for doing so are an example of how one may apply the PPS to a group.

Feedback Report

The ongoing implementation of a program plan for implementation of the PPS can also follow the format for review and revision of the program plans. In the review process, the question of outcomes is addressed followed by what may have worked in achieving those outcomes before defining the objectives for the next interim. Data are reported in relation to the overall program implementation in the same format used for reporting data about individual patients. Status of the degree of program-wide implementation is reported in relation to the level of participation achieved for the various questions addressed (status, goals, and what works) with patients. New goals for the program are described and ideas are generated from the staff as to how to improve the ways the program was being carried out.

The level of participation of the staff versus the directors can vary in respect to the several questions. For example, the new goals for the coming quarter were recommended by the director for "agreement" or "confirmed agreement" by the staff. However, the decision was to encourage the staff to participate on a higher level, hopefully at a "statement" level in answer to questions as to how the program might work more efficiently or effectively. For example, ideas arose from staff members as to the need for further training of new staff, methods for alleviating the patient's anxiety, and so forth. The aim is to generate increased commitment by attention being paid to the questions addressed by the staff and the level of participation achieved.

Table 5-11 describes the feedback report made to the program-wide team in what is called the Town Meeting Report using the same format as for individual cases in the Team Conference Report (see Table 4-2). The aim was to enhance the awareness of the staff as to the feedback report at the quarterly town meeting by using a format with which they were familiar. The same categories were used on the horizontal axis. The difference in the vertical axis was, instead of areas of disability, to use the various times when assessment of patient participation would go on. The present status of the degree of implementation is reported in accordance with the participation scale. For example, the status question was being addressed at "A" (agreement) level in 100% of the cases at the admission team conference, with a higher level of participation (84% at "A" and 16% at greater than "A" level) at the discharge team conference; and almost a reversal of those proportions at the time of the first follow-up (14% at the "A" level with 86% speaking for themselves at a "statement" level). There was a somewhat lesser albeit similar progression in participation in the status of the use of the goal question. The status of the use of "What works?" also showed a major change at the time of the follow-up visit. It is clear that the patient functioned considerably better in terms of participation at the time of follow-up than during the discharge team conference. The staff was presented this information and they were considered to be functioning in an "agreement" mode to data about the status of the program outcomes. There was greater degree of participation in answer to the question as to what might be contributing to these different results.

New goals were stated by the program director as listed: generally they were to increase the degree of participation at the admission and discharge team conferences in respect to the status question so that 50% of the patients were functioning at greater than "A" level by the time of discharge. The projected improvement in the degree of participation by the discharge conference sought in respect to the goal question was somewhat less in recognition of the lower levels of participation previously achieved. The implementation of the "What works?" question was to generate at least one to two descriptors per patient. No goal was set as to the level of participation to be achieved in respect to these descriptors. The aim was to have the staff address this question with the patient on a more consistent basis. These figures reflect some modifications contributed by the staff, hence the scale score of "CA" for "confirmed agreement."

Table 5-11. A Rehabilitation Team Conference Worksheet with the Rehabilitation Team as the Patient

What the SRP team can elicit from patients at:	Status/Progress	New Goals	What Works/Cues
Admission team conference	1 100% A for status [A] 100% A for Goals 1–2 What Works descriptors	1 Status: 75% A 25% CA/S/SS Goals: 100% A [CA]	Patient present team conference Any verbalization of goals and/or status is valuable [SS]
Discharge team conference	2 Status: 84% A 16% CA/S [A] Goals: 91% A 9% CA 2–4 What Works descriptors	2 Status: 50% A 50% CA/S/SS Goals: 75% A 25% CA/S/SS 1–2 What works descriptors/patient [CA]	Participation increases patient's sense that "They really are interested in my opinion" [S]
First follow-up visit	3 Status: 14% A 86% S/SS [A] Goals: 25% A/CA 75% S/SS What Works: 16% A/CA 86% S/SS	3 To be discussed [ ]	Small, intimate setting of doctor visit allows greater confidence to speak for themselves [S]

Participation: Asset (A), Confirmed Asset (CA), Statement (S), Specific Statement (SS)

Chapter 6
Educational Programs

THE GOALS OF THE CHAPTER

PROFESSIONAL GROWTH AND DEVELOPMENT

HAND MANAGEMENT MASTER'S DEGREE COURSE

UNDERGRADUATE ACADEMIC COURSE
Outline of an Undergraduate Course for Physical Therapy Students in Patient Participation Planning

IN-SERVICE TRAINING
In-Service Course: Patient Participation Program Planning—Occupational and Physical Therapy Departments

THE GOALS OF THE CHAPTER

This chapter continues to show the applicability of the planning questions and the steps in answering them to different educational settings in the professional life of the therapist. To learn the planning process in a group setting such as the classroom provides an opportunity for the student/therapist to experience in a personal way the same procedures eventually to be used with patients. The ultimate aim is to integrate the procedures illustrated in this book into the future professional life of the therapist. This chapter describes in detail several courses in formal academic settings as well in-service training for practitioners specifically devoted to this planning process but also how this same process can be used throughout one's career regardless of the content of the course.

PROFESSIONAL GROWTH AND DEVELOPMENT

Beginning with formal professional education, therapists are thrust into a lifelong educational process. Stimuli for this continuing education are both external and internal. External stimuli include licensure requirements, agency policies, collegial exchanges, and challenging patient cases. Internal stimuli arise from a recognition of a gap in one's knowledge, that more information on a topic is needed to feel competent.

To learn efficiently, it is helpful to use a structured process. The planning method described in this book provides such a structure. One can choose to use form PPS-1W (*W* for *weighting*), a modification of PPS-1, to explore concerns relative to the topic of interest and to select a major concern. A shared weighting procedure is used for the selection step in respect to concerns. This shared weighting procedure has been described in Chapter 2. One can then explore goals and specify a goal. Note that the levels of participation are not applicable in self-planning. The PPS-1W form illustrated in Table 6-1 adds a section for *value* of concerns, which is determined by the shared weighting process.

The following are examples of the process being used to establish learning goals. In the first situation, senior occupational therapy students were asked to submit to the instructor three topic choices for a term paper. The instructor then reviewed the topics, approved one, and returned the selected topic to each student. However, many of the students had difficulty selecting three choices to submit. Table 6-2 demonstrates the use of the planning process to arrive at a topic by one

---

Table 6-1. PPS-IW

NAME _____   DATE _____

1. **What are your concerns?**
   A.
   B.
   C.

2. **What are your major concerns?**
   Values
   A.
   B.
   C.

3. **What do you want to see happen? What would make you feel that you are making progress? What are your goals? Choose one.**
   A.
   B.
   C.

4. **What is your specific goal?**

A	B	C	D	**What?**
A	B	C	D	**Conditions?**
A	B	C	D	**Degree?**

   A = open-ended question: FREE CHOICE
   B = suggestions (3 options): MULTIPLE CHOICE
   C = recommendation (1 option): FORCED CHOICE
   D = prescription (tell what to do): NO CHOICE

---

student. Note that she arrived at a major concern of not knowing enough about diagnoses through the shared weighting process; this concern had a value of 4 for her. As a part of her specific goal, she felt that her referral in her paper to data from between 5 and 10 articles on the topic of psychosocial aspects of spinal cord injury would be a measure of having met her goal. In other cases, one might consider using 5 to 10 articles to be a means by which she might meet a goal of understanding psychosocial aspects.

In a second example, a postprofessional graduate student used the procedure as she neared the completion of her degree. The process enabled the student to identify a goal relative to future clinical work. The results are presented in Table 6-3. For two of her concerns statements, she elected to make multiple comments for the purpose of clarification. For example, she clarified in concern statement 1.B that she had a specific problem with the differential diagnosis of wrist and pain disorders. Use of these multiple comments as part of exploration may

---

Table 6-2. PPS-1W: Selection of Paper Topic

1. **What are your concerns?**
   A. Patient transfers
   B. Not knowing diagnoses well enough to intervene with patients
   C. Evaluations—time lapse since learning evaluations such as joint range of motion and muscle testing

2. **What are your major concerns?**
   Values

(2)	1	1	A. Patient transfers
(4)	2	2	B. Not knowing diagnoses well enough to intervene with patients
(3)	2	1	C. Evaluations—time lapse since learning evaluations such as joint range of motion and muscle testing

3. **What do you want to see happen? What would make you feel that you are making progress? What are your goals? Choose one.**
   A. With CVA patients, knowing where to start, what to do first, what kind of activities to use
   *B. With SCI patients, knowing where to start
   C. With head injury patients, knowing where to start

4. **What is your specific goal?**
   What?   I want to be able to discuss psychosocial aspects of spinal cord injury and its implications for occupational therapy.
   Conditions?   in a paper,
   Degree?   discussing 5–10 articles.

   Time line: November 11, paper due date

---

be helpful to a user of the process. Also, note that the student expressed four goals rather than three. Three steps of exploration are considered a reasonable minimum; more items are permissible if the person chooses.

In a third situation, a postprofessional graduate student had completed the first phase of a teaching practicum and was preparing for the second phase. To help the student prepare for the next phase, PPS-1W was used. Table 6-4 summarizes the results. Following the completion of the second and final phase, PPS-3 was used. The PPS-3 results are illustrated in Table 6-5.

You can use the planning process for your own continuing self-education. Perhaps you have to research a difficult patient case. Or perhaps you have to organize and present a department in-service

---

Table 6-3. PPS-1W: Graduate Student Interview

---

1. **What are your concerns?**
   A. Schedule of 2 patients per hour with instantaneous decisions needed; need to be able to make quick judgments
   B. Differential diagnosis; especially with pain and wrist disorders
   C. Don't trust my sensory mapping with the Semmes-Weinstein

2. **What are your major concerns?**
   Values

(5)	3		2	A. Schedule of 2 patients per hour with instantaneous decisions needed; need to be able to make quick judgments
(3)		2	1	B. Differential diagnosis; especially with pain and wrist disorders
(1)	0	1		C. Don't trust my sensory mapping with the Semmes-Weinstein

3. **What do you want to see happen? What would make you feel that you are making progress? What are your goals? Choose one.**
   *A. Less second guessing about treatment after the patient has left
   B. Less anxiety prior to patient visits
   C. Less need to consult books before making a decision
   D. Send the patient out knowing that I've done my best

4. **What is your specific goal?**
   What?   I want to use all appropriate therapeutic principles (e.g., splinting) to their optimal levels
   Conditions?   With persons with new hand injuries at the time of their first clinic visit
   Degree?   75% of the time.
   Time line: If working 20 hours/week, by February 1

---

program. Use the blank PPS-1W form provided in Table 6-1 to begin to address whatever educational concerns you have just as you have done throughout this book.

HAND MANAGEMENT MASTER'S DEGREE COURSE

The planning process was used to develop a post-professional master's degree course for students in hand management. The course focused

---

Table 6-4. PPS-IW: Preparing for Teaching Practicum

1. **What are your concerns?**
   A. Frustration over students not understanding what is being said in lecture
   B. My lecture delivery may not be interesting—too flat?
   C. I'd like to balance my presentation with handouts and other varied learning experiences.

2. **What are your major concerns?**
   Values

(4)	2		2	A. Frustration over students not understanding what is being said in lecture
(2)		1	1	B. My lecture delivery may not be interesting—too flat?
(3)	1	2		C. I'd like to balance my presentation with handouts and other varied learning experiences.

3. **What do you want to see happen? What would make you feel that you are making progress? What are your goals? Choose one.**
   A. Students will be able to do the lab exercise correctly without asking questions.
   *B. I will see that the students are doing the lab exercises correctly.
   C. Students will independently ask questions while indicating that they have integrated information.

4. **What is your specific goal?**
   What?   I would like to present the basic technique of proprioceptive neuromuscular facilitation
   Conditions?   in 2-hour lecture/labs October 18 and 20
   Degree?   so that students complete all exercises according to the guidelines established in the syllabus.

---

on three areas related to patients with hand impairments: work, leisure, and activities of daily living. By using the planning process with students to plan the course, the students not only learned about the three content areas but they experienced a process to use in practice with patients with hand impairments.

Four occupational therapists and one physical therapist were enrolled in this 3-credit course. All of the students had extensive clinical experience in hand therapy and vast knowledge of this practice area.

At the first course meeting, students were asked to come to the second class session with their concerns/interests about hand impairment

---

Table 6-5. PPS-3: Teaching Practicum

1. **What results have you achieved?**
   A. Didn't complete in 2 hours as planned but did present all I
   wanted to
   B More comfortable with using slides and overhead projector
   *C. Students followed the guidelines in the syllabus completing the
   lab exercises correctly about proprioceptive neuromuscular
   facilitation in lecture/lab on October 18 and 20.

2. **What worked?**
   A. Newness motivated them
   B. I reminded them to refer to the syllabus guidelines.
   C. Used more slides

3. **What are your concerns?**
   Values

(4)	2		2	A. Balance amount of information and time frame
(3)		2	1	B. My lecture pace was too fast.
(2)	1	1		C. Lack of immediate student feedback

4. **Goals**

   *A. Provide same content without extending beyond 2-hour limit
   B. Sense that information is presented in an integrated fashion
   C. Students performing more independently in lab

5. **What is plan?**
   Goal: Present same content on neuromuscular facilitation in
   next session within 2-hour time limit
   Means: Using 25–30 colored slides during presentation to
   graduate students depicting diagonals of motion,
   combined movements of upper and lower extremities,
   and basic procedures

   Time line: By the end of spring semester

---

and the work content area. The course instructor used the questions of concerns and goals and the steps of exploration, selection (with clustering and shared weighting), and specification in the second class session. Table 6-6 reflects the results of the initial course planning as it relates to the "work" content area.

Thirteen individual concerns/interests were elicited from the students and then clustered into four themes to make the planning manageable. For example, individual concerns 1, 2, 3, 5, and 10 have the common theme of evaluation. The students then voted to assign priority to each theme with safety/prevention at priority level 4 having the

Table 6-6. Work and Hand Rehabilitation: Initial Planning Aug. 24

What are your interests/concerns?

1. Full range of evaluations
2. Whether a given patient will be able to return to work—prognosis
3. What do evaluation results mean relative to performing a job
4. Relationships between work simulation and work
5. Safety—have doubts—how to measure relationship to impairment
6. Prevention—philosophy of safety and productivity
7. What is human potential on work force
8. What is work—value, why
9. Work as therapy
10. Job analysis
11. How does our health care system compare internationally such as workmen's compensation, health insurance, etc.
12. Psychosocial aspects of work or lack of work
13. Individual worker and society

What are your major concerns (clustered)?

Value

1 Evaluation: 1, 2, 3, 5, 10
4 Safety/prevention: 5 & 6
3 Theory of work: 4, 7, 8, 9, 12
2 Worker and society: 7, 8, 11, 13

What do you want to see happen (as a class)?

Value

3 Identify ways that we can contribute to safety and prevention as therapists
1 Describe (look at) management processes that impact on work schedules, etc.
3 Identify what factors threaten workers
2 Educate workers as to safety before work

What is the specific goal?

What? We should be able to identify hazards.

When/Where? At between 1–3 Richmond area job sites (e.g., Philip Morris, Reynolds, VCU)

Degree? Numbering 4 major hazards/site (either acute, accumulated, or direct).

Means

Each student review at least one article or book on topic and be prepared to discuss (including past experience)
Contact employer/job site
Schedule time
Gather supplies to measure and record
Visit as group
Discuss findings
Feedback to job site; plant M.D. and supervisor contacted

Time line: Nov. 21

greatest priority for course study. The students were then asked what they wanted to see happen in the course dealing with this topic of safety/prevention. They identified four general goals during exploration and selected two similar ones to be the basis for a specific goal. From the two selected general goals, the students were led through specification to develop one of the specific goals of the course.

The final stage in planning for the work content areas was to explore and decide on means to use to achieve the specific goal and a time line within the course context. A similar process was used to carry out planning for the other content areas.

UNDERGRADUATE ACADEMIC COURSE

This course dealt with the entire set of questions for undergraduate students over the length of their educational program throughout their first full year in professional school. Some assignments connected with the course were integrated into the schedule of the various types of field assignments.

Patient participation in planning was the first unit of a course entitled "Clinical Problem Solving and Communications." This course took place during the first semester for entering undergraduate physical therapy students and was generally concerned with the following goals: to provide models for clinical problem-solving, interpersonal communications, and ethical decision-making; and to discuss psychosocial issues that influence those three models. The participatory planning process is perceived to be related to all three functions.

The goals of this initial participatory planning component are to lead each student to experience the specification of concerns and goals for self, with peers, and with a patient. The unit begins with several lectures and laboratories on the two basic questions outlined in Chapter 2. It ends with the students carrying out an interview with one patient, eliciting specific goals in an area relevant to concerns, with maximal patient participation. This is critiqued by faculty and peers using a standard evaluation form (see Table 6-1). We have made several videotapes of patients being interviewed so that the students can have an example to critique using a standard scoring form (see Table 6-2). The students are introduced to the third planning question in dealing with evaluation of outcomes immediately after the completion of this first patient interview, and they set new goals for themselves. This patient interview is their first experience in clinical interaction within the entire curriculum. The class then proceeds to other topics.

We return to participatory patient planning three further times with assignments for fall and spring part-time clinical work and before their full-time summer clinical affiliation between their first and second curricular years. The goals for these later assignments are as follows. For the fall clinical rotation, the students apply the experience doing the supervised interview to two additional patients, on their own. They deal with the questions of concerns and goals in the clinical setting. The spring rotation provides an opportunity to see a patient more than once, so the students are asked to interview the same patient more than once and to ask the question about outcomes and re-evaluation of concerns and goals in the light of those outcomes. Further, they integrate the results of these interviews into the clinical record (SOAP notes or narrative). This material is incorporated in Chapter 4. The summer affiliation provides an opportunity to follow at least one patient over several weeks. The assignment from this course is for the first time to document all five questions in the format of the medical record. A detailed curricular plan for this entire program follows.

Outline of an Undergraduate Course for Physical Therapy Students or Patient Participation in Program Planning

The first part of this course can be done in about 6 weeks, with one lecture and one laboratory each week, as indicated below.

    I.   Session 1: 50 minutes (large group)
        A. Preclass activities
            1. Prepare syllabus for the course (schedule, topical outline, reading assignments, reprints, and so forth).
        B. Classroom activities
            1. Outline the entire course on clinical problem-solving and communications.
            2. Make an assignment to read the Introduction to Part One and Chapter 1 in this book.
        C. Instructional aids
            1. Textbook
            2. Course syllabus
            3. Chalkboard
   II.   Session 2: 50 minutes (large group)
        A. Preclass activities
            1. Prepare extra copies of PPS-1.
        B. Classroom activities
            1. Review and expand on instructor's concerns that led to

the development of this course and the instructor's goals for the course.

2. Ask, "What are your concerns?" Lecture, stimulate discussion of the content of assigned text, Illustrate use of the exercise at the end of Chapter 1.

3. Ask as many students as time allows to state their concerns about mastering the knowledge and skills taught in this segment of this course. Write their concerns on the board.

4. Hand out additional copies of PPS-1 and ask the students to complete it relative to their own concerns in this course, to be completed before their first laboratory. Assign Chapter 2 in the text.

C. Instructional aids
   1. Handouts (PPS-1)
   2. Chalkboard

III. Session 3: 2 hours, in groups of 10 students or less
   A. Laboratory exercise
      1. Each student states his or her chief concern from the PPS-1 forms. These concerns are written on the board, and one student acts as secretary to record on paper what is written on the board. The instructor saves this paper for use in the next laboratory.
      2. Each student then specifies (what, where or when, and degree) his or her own concern.
      3. As opportunity or need arises, instruction and examples are provided by the instructor on any course-relevant points raised by the exercise.
      4. Hand out additional copies of PPS-1 and ask the students to complete it in its entirety in terms of concerns, goals, and specificity of goals to be completed before next large group session.
   B. Instructional aids
      1. Chalkboard
      2. Paper and pencil

IV. Session 4: 50 minutes (large group)
   A. Preclass activities
      1. Prepare handout of PPS-1.
   B. Classroom activities
      1. Opportunity for students to state their concerns on previous learning activities is provided.
      2. Lecture, discuss, and illustrate content relative to goals.
      3. As time permits, write a few student-generated goals

on the board from the student's homework assignments, emphasizing specificity of goals.

    4. Discuss and illustrate differences between goals and means.

    5. Hand out a copy of PPS-1 and assign student to interview someone (e.g., relative, friend) other than a classmate using this form and to complete the concerns and goals portion of the form: due in 1 week.

  C. Instructional aids

    1. PPS-1

    2. Chalkboard

V. Session 5: 2 hours, in groups of 10 students or less

  A. Prelaboratory activities

    1. Arrange for video equipment to be in the laboratory.

    2. Evaluate PPS-1 homework assignments and return.

  B. Laboratory exercise

    1. Each student reads his or her chief concern from the record made in the first laboratory exercise. The student then states a goal for that concern, and the goal is written on the board. The student specifies his or her goal. Students are encouraged to ask for assistance from other class members, if necessary. Class members can also ask for permission to offer suggestions.

    2. A videotape of a patient interview done by one of the instructors is shown. The tape should be stopped frequently by the instructor to illustrate and discuss what is happening in the taped interview, emphasizing the levels of participation and the fact that the interviewer informed the patient of what was to happen and asked permission to move down the scale of levels of participation used in Table 2-1.

    3. As opportunity or need arises, instruction and examples should be provided by the instructor on any course-relevant points raised by the exercise.

  C. Instructional aids

    1. Chalkboard

    2. Videotaped interview

    3. Videotape player and screen

VI. Session 6: 50 minutes (large group)

  A. Preclass activities

    1. Prepare at least four copies for each student of handouts of a scoring sheet based on Table 2-1.

    2. Read and comment on PPS-1 forms from peer interviews; return through student mailboxes.

    3. Prepare a schedule for clinical interviews.

  B. Classroom activities

    1. Opportunity to express concerns on previous learning activities is provided. What outcomes were achieved? What problems remain?

    2. Lecture, discuss, and illustrate content relative to scoring interviews for levels of patient participation.

    3. Discuss the videotape quiz scheduled for next week. Hand out and discuss the scoring form.

    4. Hand out and discuss schedule of clinical interviews.

  C. Instructional aids

    1. Handouts or videotape scoring form and interview schedule.

VII. Session 7: 2 hours, with groups of 10 students or less

  A. Prelaboratory activities

    1. Arrange for videotape equipment to be in the laboratory.

    2. Arrange to place videotapes in media library for student use.

  B. Laboratory exercise

    1. A videotape of an interview done by an instructor is viewed with frequent interruptions to discuss level of patient participation illustrated in the interview. Students score.

    2. Students view a second taped interview and score without interruption. Students then compare their scoring efforts, and the laboratory project is discussed.

    3. Students are offered the opportunity to study videotapes of interviews in the media library of the university.

  C. Instructional aids

    1. Scoring forms for video interviews (Table 6-7)

    2. Videotapes of two interviews

    3. Video equipment

VIII. Session 8: 30 minutes (large group), videotape quiz.

  A. Preclass activities

    1. Have available a videotaped interview that the students have not seen.

    2. Prepare handouts of patient participation scoring forms.

    3. Arrange for videotape viewing equipment to be in the classroom.

Table 6-7. Scoring Form for Analysis of Videotapes

The Therapist	1	2	3	4	5	6	7	8	9	10	11	12	13	14	15
A. Asks open-ended questions without suggesting answers	16	17	18	19	20	21	22	23	24	25	26	27	28	29	30
B. Suggests 3 options/answers															
C. Recommends 1 option/answer															
D. Tells what to do															
E. Reflection and other															
A. Asks open-ended questions without suggesting answers															
B. Suggests 3 options/answers															
C. Recommends 1 option/answer															
D. Tells what to do															
E. Reflection and other															

  B. Classroom activities
   1. Hand out patient participation scoring forms.
   2. Show videotaped interview for students to score.
  C. Instructional aids
   1. Videotaped interview
   2. Videotape-viewing equipment
   3. Scoring forms
  D. Postquiz activity
   1. Grade quiz and report scores to students in some
    appropriate way.
 IX. Session 9: 45 minutes for *each* student, in groups of three or
  four students per instructor
  A. Preclinical activity
   1. Prepare sufficient copies of form PPS-1.
   2. Prepare sufficient copies of form found in Table 6-8.
   3. Schedule patients and students.
  B. Clinical activities
   1. Each student interviews a patient, working from PPS-1
    to obtain all information required by that form.
   2. Other students and instructor fill out form from
    Table 6-8.
   3. Interviewing student critiques himself or herself and
    discusses his or her interview.
   4. Each observing student provides feedback to the inter-
    viewing student concerning his or her performance
    during the interview.
   5. The instructor provides feedback to the interviewing
    student and makes such other instructional points as
    may have been illustrated during the interview. The
    interviews are not graded because our experience indi-
    cates that grading creates such anxiety that little learn-
    ing occurs.

  The nine sessions outlined above constitute a unit within the year-
long course on clinical problem-solving and communications. It occu-
pies about 6 weeks. Other units are taken up in sequence after session
9. The following sessions are interspersed at appropriate times during
the year.
 X. Session 10: fall part-time clinical experience
  A. Assignment: 15 minutes (large group)
   1. Students are given form PPS-2 and asked to fill it out
    and hand it in to the instructor before beginning the
    fall clinical rotation of a half a day per week for

Table 6-8. Interview Evaluation Form: Patient Participation in Planning for Therapy

	Not Attempted	Attempted		Comments
		Incomplete	Complete	
1. Did interviewer:				
A. Introduce patient to overall procedures?				
B. Introduce exploration of concerns?				
C. Elicit at least 3 concerns?				
D. Ask for selection of priorities (either shared weights or priority)?				
E. Confirm major concern(s)?				
F. Introduce exploration of goals?				
G. Introduce cooperative role in identifying goals?				
H. Elicit 3 goals?				
I. Ask for selection of one goal to pursue?				
J. Specify goal: what?				
K. setting?				
L. degree?				

2. Did interview start with open-ended question?

_____

3. Did interviewer ask patient's consent before moving to multiple choice, forced choice, or prescription?

_____

4. Did student move down steps in correct order?

_____

5. Did student return to open-ended questions at an appropriate time?

_____

2 weeks. It is to be completed in regard to their own accomplishments, remaining concerns and goals in completing their own learning or knowledge, and skills relative to the content of this book.

B. Preclinical activities

1. Critique student forms PPS-2 in terms of threefold exploration and specification of selected outcomes, concerns, and goals. Return to students prior to their clinical rotation.

2. Hand out form PPS-1 and assign students to complete the form with at least 1 patient during their fall clinical rotation and turn it in to the instructor.

C. Postclinical activities

1. Critique student forms PPS-1 done during the clinical rotation with particular emphasis on relevance of goals to selected main concern, adequate exploration of goals, specification of selected goal, and level of partic-ipation. Return them to students.

XI. Session 11: spring part-time clinical experience

A. Assignment: 15 minutes (large group)

1. Students are given form PPS-3 and asked to fill it out and hand it in to the instructor before beginning the spring clinical rotation of 1 full day per week for 2 weeks. It is to be completed in regard to their own concerns in completing their learning or knowledge and skills relative to the content of this book.

2. Read Chapter 3 in textbook.

B. Preclinical activities

1. Critique student forms PPS-3 and return to students before their clinical rotation.

2. Hand out forms PPS-1 and PPS-2 and assign students to complete both the initial and follow-up forms with a patient during their spring clinical rotation and to turn it in to the instructor. Hand in copies of their clinical SOAP notes containing material relevant to this course.

3. Discuss in class the content of Chapter 3, emphasizing the question of outcomes. (15 minutes [large group])

C. Postclinical activities

1. Critique student forms and SOAP notes written during the clinical rotation with same emphasis as in the fall clinical rotation and return them to students.

XII. Session 12: summer full-time clinical affiliation

A. Assignment: 15 minutes (large group)

    1. Students are given form PPS-3 and asked to fill it out and hand in to the instructor before beginning the summer clinical rotation. It is to be completed in regard to their own concerns in completing their learning or knowledge and skills relative to the content of this book.

    2. Read Chapter 4 in textbook.

B. Preclinical activities

    1. Critique student forms PPS-3, which should be complete in every respect, and return to students prior to their clinical rotation.

    2. Discuss in class the content of Chapter 4, emphasizing the question of what worked. (30 minutes [large group])

    3. Assign the students to hand in at the end of the summer one SOAP note (or whatever format is used in the clinic where they work). This copy of the clinical record is to demonstrate the answering of all five questions posed in the Introduction to Part One to this text. It must, therefore, represent at least three evaluative sessions with the patient.

C. Postclinical activities

    1. Critique student SOAP notes or other documentation done during the clinical rotation and return to students.

IN-SERVICE TRAINING

A short-term course for physical and occupational therapists in a large medical center used the planning process as a basis for its organization as well as for its content. The staff supervisors felt that there was a need for the staff to meet the requirements of accreditation agencies to incorporate patients into the planning process to a greater degree. Still other issues dealt with staff burnout and the need to develop new formats for working with the large variety of patients, particularly those with cognitive impairments. The concerns of the therapists themselves have been illustrated earlier in Table 5-8. They formed the basis for the design of the course to be described.

    The course lasted 7 hours and was implemented in conjunction with the daily duties of the therapists and was applied in their own work. Once the therapists had experienced the first two questions as to concerns and goals and the awareness of the levels of participation, they put these several questions to work with patients.

By the end of the course, the classroom sessions had dealt with the entire set of questions. Once the therapists had experienced the use of the questions in the classroom, they then applied them to their work with patients. Emphasis was primarily on the steps of exploration, selection, and specification and levels of participation as exemplified in any one or several of the questions. The specific goals of each of the sessions, the procedures followed, and the evaluation of results are described in detail as follows.

In-Service Course: Patient Participation in Program Planning—Occupational and Physical Therapy Departments

Instructor's Course Goal (Outcome)

What: Participants will be able to generate outcome statements, solution statements, need statements, and goal statements.

When/where: During the course of ongoing therapeutic relationship daily or as needed

Degree: Meeting the criteria of specificity, relevance, and fit as appropriate for the content of the statements.

Time line: At the end of session 5

Preassignment

Exploration of concerns and selection using form PPS-1. Optional reading assignment is Introduction to Part One and Chapters 1 and 2 of textbook. Distribute 1 week prior to session 1.

  I. Session 1: 75 minutes, required of all staff
    A. Content and activities; emphasis is experiential learning
      1. Explore concerns as a large group and briefly discuss exploration after all concerns are generated based on preassignment.
      2. Discuss selection and shared weighting technique. Have participants perform shared weighting on three concerns generated during group.
      3. Introduce and discuss goals. Have participants generate three general goal statements for major concern identified through shared weighting.

4. Introduce and discuss goal specification. Have participants choose one general goal and specify.
5. At conclusion
   a. Collect preassignments and goal statements generated during session.
   b. Announce tentative schedule for remaining sessions and voluntary participation. Registration procedures for remaining sessions.

B. Instructional aids
   1. Easel pad
   2. Marking pens
   3. Masking tape
   4. Chalkboard

C. Instructor activities between sessions 1 and 2
   1. Review participants' preassignments and goal statements. Critique and return.
   2. Identify three clusters from participants' goal statements.
   3. Complete PPS-1G (PPS-2 or PPS-3).
   4. Prepare handout for session 2 that indicates goal clusters, instructor's short-term goals, and tentative remaining schedule.

II. Session 2: 90 minutes
A. Instructor's short-term goal
   1. What: Participants will be able to write a specific goal relevant to expressed concerns.
   2. Where/when: During class
   3. Degree: So that goal meets requirements of specification
   4. Time line: By the completion of session 2

B. Content and activities
   1. Provide copies of all handouts or refer to tables in text (see Tables 2-2 to 2-8).
      a. Participants' and instructor's goals and tentative schedule
      b. PPS-1
      c. Patient participation scale (see Table 2-1)
   2. Review goal/schedule handout, which includes clusters of course goals generated from participants.
      a. Effectively involve patients with cognitive difficulties in treatment.
      b. Motivate patients.
      c. Set realistic goals.

     3. Participants individually complete PPS-1 relative to homework assignment 1 of interviewing patients.

     4. Group discusses PPS responses.

     5. Introduce and discuss patient participation scale.

     6. Show videotape of interview and have participants evaluate outcomes achieved relative to their goals for impending patient interviews.

     7. At conclusion

        a. Collect individual program planning sheets.

        b. Review homework assignment; distribute extra program planning sheets.

   C. Instructional aids

     1. Handouts

     2. Easel pad

     3. Masking tape

     4. Marker pens

     5. Videotape

     6. Videotape player and monitor

     7. Chalkboard

   D. Instructor activities between sessions 2 and 3

     1. Review collected materials.

     2. Complete PPS-2 or PPS-3.

Homework Assignment 1

Review book section that distinguishes between goals and means; conduct at least two patient interviews using PPS-1. Read Chapter 3 of textbook.

   III.   Session 3: 90 minutes

     A. Instructor's short-term goal

        1. What: Participants will be able to identify results/outcomes relative to their practice with patients

        2. When/where: From current clinical case load

        3. Degree: So that they can list at least three outcomes with the best outcome stated to meet the four criteria of specificity

        4. Time line: by the completion of homework assignment 2

     B. Content and activities

        1. Review instructor's goal from session 2 and homework assignment. What did participants accomplish?

        a. Write a specific goal relevant to the patient's concern.

       b. State level of patient participation in defining patient goals.

    2. Introduce today's goal—outcomes and new form.

       a. List three outcomes for *your* use of the planning process.

       b. Select most important outcome.

       c. Specify most important outcome.

       d. Establish time line.

       e. Use documentation; handout of examples using SOAP format.

    3. Have participants address their concerns now.

    4. At conclusion

       a. Collect forms completed by participants during class.

       b. Review homework assignment 2 and distribute necessary forms.

  C. Instructional aids

    1. Handouts

    2. Easel pad

    3. Masking tape

    4. Marking pens

  D. Instructor activities between sessions 3 and 4

    1. Review participants' assignments. Critique and return.

    2. Complete PPS-2 or PPS-3.

Homework Assignment 2

1. Follow-up interviews with three patients; if last week's patients are available, explore outcomes of last week's goals.

2. Schedule 1 of these interviews with one of the instructors as an observer.

3. Use either PPS-1 or PPS-2, as appropriate, and hand in at interview with observer.

4. Bring copies of SOAP notes to next class to hand in.

5. Review Chapter 4 in textbook.

  V. Session 4: 90 minutes

    A. Goals

      1. Instructor's short-term goals with emphasis on personalization

      2. Participant's goal of involving cognitively impaired

    B. Content and activities

1. Have participants address the following questions relative to homework assignment 2 (emphasize personalization).
   a. What outcomes were achieved?
   b. What worked?
   c. What concerns?
   d. What goals?
2. Discuss application to cognitively impaired.
3. At conclusion, review homework assignment 3.

C. Instructional aids
   1. Easel pad
   2. Masking tape
   3. Marking pens

D. Instructor: complete PPS-2 or PPS-3.

Homework Assignment 3

Conduct daily interaction with patients as to what worked, what are the goals, what worked, and so forth, which is integral to the therapeutic setting. Write logs.

V. Session 5: 60 minutes
    A. Review of course—patient as an independent problem solver

REFERENCES

1. DiMatteo MR, DiNicola DD: *Achieving Patient Compliance.* New York: Pergamon Press; 1982.

2. Dishman BK, Ickes W, Morgan WP: Self-motivation and adherence to habitual physical activity. *J Appl Soc Psychol* 10:115, 1980.

3. Care GRF, Harfield B, Chamberlain MA: And have you done your exercises? *Physiotherapy* 67:180, 1981.

4. Allen VR: Follow-up study of wrist-driven flexor hinge splint use. *AJOT* 24:420, 1971.

5. Feinberg J, Brandt HD: Use of resting splints by patients with rheumatoid arthritis. *AJOT* 35:173, 1981.

6. Seeger MS, Fisher LA: Adaptive equipment used in the rehabilitation of two arthroplasty patients. *AJOT* 36:503, 1982.

7. Sluijs EM, Kok GJ, Zee J: Correlates of exercise compliance in physical therapy. *Phys Ther* 73:771, 1993.

8. Coy JA: Autonomy-based informed consent: ethical implications for patient noncompliance. *Phys Ther* 69:826, 1989.

9. Windom PA: *The Preparedness of the Patient to Play an Active Role in Physical Therapy in the Rehabilitation Setting.* Unpublished master's thesis, Virginia Commonwealth University, 1979.

10. Taylor DP: Treatment goals for quadriplegic and paraplegic patients. *AJOT* 28:22, 1974.

11. Tresolini CP and the Pew-Fetzer Task Force: *Health Professions Education and Relationship-Centered Care.* San Francisco: Pew Health Professions Commission; 1994:9.

12. Smith TC, Thompson TL: The inherent, powerful therapeutic value of a good physician-patient relationship. *Psychosomatics* 34:166, 1993.

13. Nelson AL: Patients' perspectives of a spinal cord injury unit. *SCI Nursing* 7:44, 1990.

14. McEwen I, Shelden M: *Functional Outcomes of Physical Therapy for Children and Adults with Developmental and Acquired Disabilities.* Paper presented at the Annual Conference of the American Physical Therapy Association, Cincinnati, OH, June 13, 1993.

15. Borkan JM, Quirk M, Sullivan M: Finding meaning after the fall: injury narratives from elderly hip fracture patients. *Soc Sci Med* 33:947, 1991.

16. Borkan JM, Reis S, Hermont D, Biderman A: Talking about the pain: a patient-centered study of low-back pain in primary care. *Soc Sci Med* 40:177, 1995.

17. Ozer MN: *The Management of Persons with Spinal Cord Injury.* New York: Demos Publications; 1988:Chap 1.

18. Matheson LN: *Work Capacity Evaluation.* Anaheim, CA: Employment Rehabilitation Institute of California; 1987:1–11.

19. Nagi SZ: Some conceptual issues in disability and rehabilitation. In Sussman MB (ed): *Sociology and Rehabilitation.* Washington DC: US Department of Health, Education and Welfare; 1965:Chap 5.

20. Napier J: *Hands.* New York: Pantheon Books; 1980:23–24.

21. Doak CC, Doak LG, Root JH: *Teaching Patients with Low Literacy Skills.* Philadelphia: Lippincott; 1985.

22. Payton OD, Nelson CE, Hobbs MS: *Descriptive Study of Patients' Perceptions of Their Role in Therapy and the Roles of Health Care Providers.* Poster presentation, World Confederation for Physical Therapy, Washington, DC, June 1995.

23. Rogers JC, Figone JJ: Psychosocial parameters in treating the person with quadriplegia. *AJOT* 33:432, 1979.

24. Carpenter C: The experience of spinal cord injury: the individual's perspective-implications for rehabilitation practice. *Phys Ther* 74:614, 1994.

25. *Evaluative Criteria for Accreditation of Educational Programs for the Preparation of Physical Therapists.* Alexandria, VA: Commission of Accreditation in Physical Therapy Education, American Physical Therapy Association, 1996.

26. Purtilo RB, Meier RH: Team challenges: regulatory constraints and patient empowerment. *Am J Phys Med Rehabil* 72:327, 1993.

27. American Physical Therapy Association: Standards of practice for physical therapy and the accompanying criteria. *Phys Ther* 77:102, 1997.

28. Payton OD, Nelson CE: Involving patients in decision making. *PT, Magazine of PT* 3:74, 1995.

29. *Essentials and Guidelines for an Accredited Educational Program for the Occupational Therapist.* Bethesda, MD: American Occupational Therapy Association; 1991.

30. *Standards of Practice for Occupational Therapy.* Rockville, MD: American Occupational Therapy Association; 1991.

31. *The Psychosocial Core of Occupational Therapy.* Rockville, MD: American Occupational Therapy Association; 1995.

32. Branch WT, Arky RA, Woo B: Teaching medicine as a human experience: a patient-doctor relationship course for faculty and first-year medical students. *Ann Intern Med* 114:482, 1991.

33. Reiser SJ: The era of the patient: using the experience of illness in shaping the missions of health care. *JAMA* 269:1012, 1993.

34. Gluekauf RL: Use and misuse of assessment in rehabilitation: getting back to basics. In Gluekauf RL, Sechrest RB, Bond GR, McConel EG (eds): *Improving Assessment in Rehabilitation and Health.* Newbury Park, CA: Sage Publications; 1993.

35. Wax TM: Matchmaking among cultures: disability culture and the larger marketplace. In Gluekauf RL, Sechrest RB, Bond GR, McConel EG (eds): *Improving Assessment in Rehabilitation and Health.* Newbury Park, CA: Sage Publications; 1993.

36. Bacharach SB: Organizational theories: some criteria for evaluation. *Acad Manage Rev* 14:496, 1989.

37. Kerlinger F: *Foundations of Behavioral Research* 3rd ed. Fort Worth: Harcourt, Brace, Jovanovich; 1996.

38. Engel GL: The need for a new medical model: a challenge for biomedicine. *Science* 196:129, 1977.

39. Engel GL: The clinical application of the biopsychosocial model. *Am J Psychiatry* 137:535, 1980.

40. Sadler JZ, Hulgus YF: Clinical problem solving and the biopsychosocial model. *Am J Psychiatry* 149:1315, 1992.

41. Waddlee G: A new clinical model for the treatment of low back pain. *Spine* 12:632, 1987.

42. Dworkin SF, Massoth DL: Temporamandibular disorders and chronic pain: disease or illness? *J Prosthet Dent* 72:29, 1994.

43. Dean E: Psychobiological adaptation model for physical therapy practice. *Phys Ther* 65:1061, 1985.

44. Ashworth PD, Longmate MA, Morrison P: Patient participation: its meaning and significance in the context of caring. *J Adv Nurs* 17:1430, 1992.

45. Smith RC, Hoppe RB: The patient's story: integrating the patient and physician-centered approaches to interviewing. *Ann Intern Med* 115:470, 1991.

46. Gerteis M, Edgman-Levitan S et al (eds): *Through the Patient's Eyes: Understanding and Promoting Patient-Centered Care.* San Francisco: Jossey-Bass; 1993.

47. Ellers B: Involving and supporting family and friends. In Gerteis M, Edgman-Levitan S et al (eds): *Through the Patient's Eyes: Understanding and Promoting Patient-Centered Care.* San Francisco: Jossey Bass; 1993.

48. DiMatteo MR, DiNicola DD: Norms and compliance: the effect of the patient's culture. In DiMatteo DM, DiNicola DD (eds): *Achieving Patient Compliance.* New York: Pergamon Press; 1982.

49. Edgman-Levitan S: Providing effective emotional support. In Gerteis M, Edgman-Levitan S et al (eds): *Through the Patient's Eyes: Understanding and Promoting Patient-Centered Care.* San Francisco: Jossey-Bass; 1993.

50. Allshouse KD: Treating patients as individuals. In Gerteis M, Edgman-Levitan S et al (eds): *Through the Patient's Eyes: Understanding and Promoting Patient-Centered Care.* San Francisco: Jossey-Bass; 1993.

51. Kaplan SH, Greenfield S, Ware JE: Assessing the effects of physician-patient interactions on the outcomes of chronic disease. *Med Care* 27:S110, 1989.

52. Roberson MHB: The meaning of compliance: patient perspectives. *Qualitative Health Research* 2:7, 1992.

53. Sluijs EM, Kok GJ, Zee J: Correlates of exercise compliance in physical therapy. *Phys Ther* 73:771, 1993.

54. DiMatteo MR, DiNicola DD: The compliance problem: an introduction. In DiMatteo MR, DiNicola DD (eds): *Achieving Patient Compliance.* New York: Pergamon Press; 1982.

55. Delblanco TL: Promoting the doctor's involvement in care. In Gerteis M, Edgman-Levitan S et al (eds): *Through the Patient's Eyes: Understanding and Promoting Patient-Centered Care.* San Francisco: Jossey-Bass; 1993.

56. Moloney TW, Paul B: Rebuilding public trust and confidence. In Gerteis M, Edgman-Levitan S et al (eds): *Through the Patient's Eyes: Understanding and Promoting Patient-Centered Care.* San Francisco: Jossey-Bass; 1993.

57. Greenfield S, Kaplan S, Ware JE: Expanding patient involvement in care: effects on patient outcomes. *Ann Intern Med* 102:520, 1985.

58. Malzer RL: Patient performance level during inpatient physical rehabilitation: therapist, nurse and patient perspective. *Arch Phys Med Rehabil* 69:363, 1988.

59. Waterworth S, Luker KA: Reluctant collaborators: do patients want to be involved in decisions concerning care? *J Adv Nurs* 15:971, 1990.

60. Biley FC: Some determinants that affect patient participation in decision making about nursing care. *J Adv Nurs* 17:414, 1992.

61. Strull WM, Lo B, Charles G: Do patients want to participate in medical decision making? *JAMA* 252:2990, 1984.

62. Payton OD, Nelson CE: A preliminary study of patients' perceptions of certain aspects of their physical therapy experience. *Physiotherapy Theory and Practice* 12:27, 1996.

63. Payton OD, Nelson CE, Hobbs MSC: Physical therapy patients' perceptions of their relationships with health care professionals. *Physiotherapy Theory and Practice* 14:211, 1998.

64. Chiou IL, Burnett CN: Values of activities of daily living: a survey of stroke patients and their home therapists. *Phys Ther* 65:901, 1985.

65. Brody DS, Miller SM, Lerman CE et al: Patient perception of involvement in medical care: relationship to illness attitudes and outcomes. *J Gen Intern Med* 4:506, 1989.

66. Nelson CE, Payton OD: The planning process in occupational therapy: perceptions of adult rehabilitation patients. *AJOT* 51:576, 1997.

67. Northern JG, Rust DM, Nelson CE, Watts JH: Involvement of adult rehabilitation patients in setting occupational therapy goals. *AJOT* 29:214, 1995.

68. Payton OD, Ivey JE: The role of psychoeducation in allied health practice and education. *J Allied Health* 10:91, 1981.

69. Martin JE, Tubbert PM: Behavioral management strategies for improving health and fitness. *J Cardiac Rehabil* 4.200, 1984.

70. Sluijs EM, Zee J, Kok GJ: Differences between physical therapists in attention paid to patient education. *Physiotherapy Theory and Practice* 9:103, 1993.

71. DeMatteo MR, DiNicola DD: Practitioner-patient relationships: the communication of information. In DeMatteo MR, DiNicola DD (eds): *Achieving Patient Compliance.* New York: Pergamon Press; 1982.

72. Gagne RM, Briggs LJ, Wager WW: *Principles of Instructional Design,* 3rd ed. Chicago: Holt Rinehart Winston; 1988.

73. Trombly CA: *Occupational Therapy for Physical Dysfunction,* 2nd ed. Baltimore: Williams & Wilkins; 1983.

74. Wood PH, Bailey EM: *People with Disabilities.* New York: World Rehabilitation Fund; 1980.

INDEX

Note: Page numbers followed by *t* indicate tables.

ISBN 0-07-077882-5

90000

9 780070 778825